Update on Otorhinolaryngologic Diseases (2nd Edition)

Update on Otorhinolaryngologic Diseases (2nd Edition)

Guest Editors

Se Hwan Hwang
Do Hyun Kim

MDPI

Basel • Beijing • Wuhan • Barcelona • Belgrade • Novi Sad • Cluj • Manchester

Guest Editors

Se Hwan Hwang
Otolaryngology-Head and Neck Surgery
Bucheon St. Mary's Hospital
College of Medicine
The Catholic University of Korea
Seoul
Republic of Korea

Do Hyun Kim
Otolaryngology-Head and Neck Surgery
Seoul St. Mary's Hospital
College of Medicine
The Catholic University of Korea
Seoul
Republic of Korea

Editorial Office
MDPI AG
Grosspeteranlage 5
4052 Basel, Switzerland

This is a reprint of the Special Issue, published open access by the journal *Medicina* (ISSN 1648-9144), freely accessible at: https://www.mdpi.com/journal/medicina/special_issues/U64XMJCS7U.

For citation purposes, cite each article independently as indicated on the article page online and as indicated below:

Lastname, A.A.; Lastname, B.B. Article Title. *Journal Name* **Year**, *Volume Number*, Page Range.

ISBN 978-3-7258-4477-7 (Hbk)
ISBN 978-3-7258-4478-4 (PDF)
https://doi.org/10.3390/books978-3-7258-4478-4

Contents

About the Editors vii

Antonella Loperfido, Davide Rizzo, Bruno Fionda, Luca Mureddu, Andrea Tondo, Luca Tagliaferri, et al.
The Potential Role of the Microbiome in the Pathogenesis of Nasal Tumors: A Comprehensive Review
Reprinted from: *Medicina* **2024**, *60*, 1808, https://doi.org/10.3390/medicina60111808 1

Rasads Misirovs, Anna Kamusella, Michael Miller and Samit Majumdar
Underlying Diagnosis of Food Bolus Obstruction Acute Admissions to Otorhinolaryngology: A Shift to Provide the Best Care as per the Current Guidelines
Reprinted from: *Medicina* **2025**, *61*, 1047, https://doi.org/10.3390/medicina61061047 13

Cihan Türker, Elif Emre, Süleyman Aydın, Mustafa Dalgıç and Deniz Baklacı
An Important Biomarker in Patients with Bell's Palsy: Serum Calprotectin
Reprinted from: *Medicina* **2025**, *61*, 747, https://doi.org/10.3390/medicina61040747 22

Matthew Min Xian Yii, Antonia Rowson, Milan van Ammers and Jessica Prasad
Flexible Nasendoscopy in Stevens–Johnson Syndrome/Toxic Epidermal Necrolysis: A Ten-Year Otolaryngology Experience
Reprinted from: *Medicina* **2025**, *61*, 513, https://doi.org/10.3390/medicina61030513 30

Hyun-Il Shin, Hyunsu Choi, Jae-Kyun Jung and Choung-Soo Kim
The Modulation of Fibrosis in Vocal Fold Repair: A Study on c-Met Agonistic Antibodies and Hepatocyte Growth in Animal Studies
Reprinted from: *Medicina* **2024**, *60*, 2033, https://doi.org/10.3390/medicina60122033 37

Nicola Lombardo, Aurelio D'Ecclesia, Emanuela Chiarella, Corrado Pelaia, Debbie Riccelli, Annamaria Ruzza, et al.
Real-World Evaluation of Dupilumab in the Long-Term Management of Eosinophilic Chronic Rhinosinusitis with Nasal Polyps: A Focus on IL-4 and IL-13 Receptor Blockade
Reprinted from: *Medicina* **2024**, *60*, 1996, https://doi.org/10.3390/medicina60121996 46

Dan Bi Park, David W. Jang, Do Hyun Kim and Sung Won Kim
Development of a New Swine Model Resembling Human Empty Nose Syndrome
Reprinted from: *Medicina* **2024**, *60*, 1559, https://doi.org/10.3390/medicina60101559 58

Ji-Young Kang, Hyunsu Choi, Jeong-Min Oh, Minsu Kim and Dong-Chang Lee
$PM_{2.5}$ Induces Pyroptosis via Activation of the ROS/NF-κB Signaling Pathway in Bronchial Epithelial Cells
Reprinted from: *Medicina* **2024**, *60*, 1434, https://doi.org/10.3390/medicina60091434 71

Andrea Frosolini, Valeria Caragli, Giulio Badin, Leonardo Franz, Patrizia Bartolotta, Andrea Lovato, et al.
Optimal Timing and Treatment Modalities of Arytenoid Dislocation and Subluxation: A Meta-Analysis
Reprinted from: *Medicina* **2025**, *61*, 92, https://doi.org/10.3390/medicina61010092 84

Yun Jin Kang, Gulnaz Stybayeva and Se Hwan Hwang
Effect of the BiZact™ Low-Temperature Dissecting Device on Intra- and Postoperative Morbidities Related to Tonsillectomy—A Systematic Review and Meta-Analysis
Reprinted from: *Medicina* **2024**, *60*, 1415, https://doi.org/10.3390/medicina60091415 97

About the Editors

Se Hwan Hwang

Se Hwan Hwang works as a professor in the Department of Otolaryngology at Bucheon St. Mary's Hospital, The Catholic University of Korea. His interests include rhinology-related tissue engineering and regenerative medicine. He is a member of the Korean Society of Rhinology and Korean Tissue Engineering and the Regenerative Medicine Society.

Do Hyun Kim

Do Hyun Kim is a faculty member in the Department of Otolaryngology at Seoul St. Mary's Hospital, The Catholic University of Korea. His primary research interests include airway regeneration, olfactory regeneration, organoid technology, atrophic rhinitis, and skull base surgery. Dr. Kim serves as Editor-in-Chief of the *Journal of Rhinology* and as an Associate Editor for *Clinical and Experimental Otorhinolaryngology*. He also holds board memberships of the Korean Society of Rhinology and the Korean Society of Endoscopic Neurosurgery, and is a member of the Korean Tissue Engineering and Regenerative Medicine Society.

medicina

MDPI

Review

The Potential Role of the Microbiome in the Pathogenesis of Nasal Tumors: A Comprehensive Review

Antonella Loperfido [1], Davide Rizzo [2,3], Bruno Fionda [4,*], Luca Mureddu [2,3], Andrea Tondo [2,3], Luca Tagliaferri [4,5], Gianluca Bellocchi [1], Giovanni Delogu [6,7] and Francesco Bussu [2,3]

1 Otolaryngology Unit, San Camillo Forlanini Hospital, 00152 Rome, Italy; aloperfido@scamilloforlanini.rm.it (A.L.)
2 Otolaryngology Division, Azienda Ospedaliera Universitaria di Sassari, 07100 Sassari, Italy
3 Department of Medicine Surgery and Pharmacy, Sassari University, 07100 Sassari, Italy
4 UOC Degenze di Radioterapia Oncologica, Dipartimento di Diagnostica per Immagini e Radioterapia Oncologica, Fondazione Policlinico Universitario A. Gemelli IRCCS, 00168 Rome, Italy
5 Istituto di Radiologia, Università Cattolica del Sacro Cuore, 00168 Rome, Italy
6 Dipartimento di Scienze Biotecnologiche di Base, Cliniche Intensivologiche e Perioperatorie-Sezione di Microbiologia, Università Cattolica del Sacro Cuore, 00168 Rome, Italy
7 Mater Olbia Hospital, 07026 Olbia, Italy
* Correspondence: bruno.fionda@policlinicogemelli.it

Abstract: Cancers of the nose, and especially the nose vestibule, represent a significant challenge for clinicians due to their rarity, the intricate nature of surrounding vital structures, the nonspecific early symptoms, and the etiological factors that are not completely understood. Emerging research suggests that alterations in the nasal microbiome, also known as microbial dysbiosis, may contribute to the pathogenesis of those malignancies through mechanisms involving chronic inflammation, immune modulation, and cellular changes. The aims of this paper are to review the current literature covering the nasal microbiome's role in carcinogenesis, particularly in the context of squamous cell carcinoma, and to explore how microbial dysbiosis might foster a pro-tumorigenic environment. It further discusses potential future directions for research and therapeutic approaches.

Keywords: nasal tumors; squamous cell carcinoma; SCC; nasal vestibule; paranasal sinuses; microbiome; dysbiosis; Human Papilloma Virus; HPV; carcinogenesis

1. Introduction

Primary malignancies of the nasal cavity and paranasal sinuses are rare, accounting for less than 3% of cancers of the upper aerodigestive tract, and less than 0.5% of all cancers [1]. They pose a significant challenge for clinicians, not only due to their rarity but also because of the nonspecific early symptoms, the great variety of histological types, and the complex anatomy, which, depending on the different subsites, deeply influences patterns of spread and ultimately the therapeutic approach and prognosis. Moreover, the main potential causes and risk factors are not completely understood. Various malignant neoplasms can develop in the nasal cavity and paranasal sinuses, with the most common being squamous cell carcinoma (SCC) and adenocarcinoma variants, followed by neuroendocrine tumors and mucosal melanoma. Sinonasal SCC encompasses a broad range of tumors with diverse biological characteristics, as indicated by its genetic similarities to other sinonasal cancers, including sinonasal undifferentiated carcinoma (SNUC) and neuroendocrine carcinoma (NEC). Of these tumors, SCC, although not as predominant as in the other head and neck sites, is probably still the most frequent type identified on histology [2]. In the detection of SCC of the nose, it is essential to specify and distinguish between those affecting the nasal cavities and paranasal sinuses and those originating from the nasal vestibule. The latter have recently been a focus of interest, as the need for the standardization of definition, classification, and treatment approach has clearly emerged. At present, the AJCC staging criteria for the primary lesion (T) in the nasal vestibule are the same as those for the nasal cavity proper and the ethmoid sinus [3–5]. Therefore, the current shared international staging system does not take into account the anatomical features of these different regions and the particular spread pattern of the different tumors. According to the literature, SCC of the nasal vestibule is also considered rare among the nasal and paranasal malignancies, with an estimated annual incidence of 0.41 cases per 100,000 people and accounts for approximately 1% of all head and neck cancers. However, this prevalence might be greatly underestimated because no specific topographic WHO code exists that allows for proper retrieval from the cancer registries, and also because of the common misdiagnosis with skin primaries [6]. This can lead to deferred treatment and a consequent deterioration of survival rates [7,8].

The definition of clear radiological anatomic boundaries, and consequently a specific WHO topographic code, is a prerequisite to allow proper assessment of the real incidence. Clinicians' awareness of the possibility of a vestibule malignancy primary diagnosis should lead to recommending an endoscopic evaluation to exclude an origin inside the nasal vestibule in all SCCs arising around the nostril [9].

The incidence of nasal vestibule SCC peaks in the seventh decade of life, with a mean age between 67 and 71 years, and with a slightly higher occurrence in men. Typically, patients may refer to pain in the nasal vestibule, nasal obstruction, irritative symptoms like a burning sensation in the nose, and bleeding. Regarding risk factors, several trigger agents have been proposed including smoking, sunlight exposure, blackboard chalk typically used by teachers, and viral agents such as Human Papilloma Virus (HPV) and Epstein–Barr Virus (EBV), but the precise role of each remains contested [10].

Non-vestibular sinonasal SCC (mainly arising from the maxillary sinus, nasal cavity proper, and ethmoid) is a rare and aggressive malignancy arising from the epithelial cells lining the nasal cavity and paranasal sinuses. It has an annual incidence of about 1 in 100,000 people in most developed countries, accounting for less than 1% of all cancers and less than 4% of those originating in the head and neck area [11]. The low absolute risk in the general population has been associated with a high relative risk for specific chemical exposures and occupational environments, including woodworking, exposure to leather dust, formaldehyde, glues, nickel, chrome, arsenic and welding fumes, the textile industry, hairdressers and rubber workers [12,13]. Similarly to nasal vestibule SCC, this entity primarily affects men aged 50–70, with a male-to-female ratio of 2:1 [14]. Although environmental exposures, including wood and leather dust, tobacco smoke, HPV, and certain occupational hazards, have been identified as risk factors, the evidence on the matter is inconclusive, and the pathogenesis of sinonasal SCC remains largely unclear [15]. Another phenomenon described in the literature is the association between sinonasal SCC and inverted sinonasal papilloma [16]. Moreover, as reported for nasal vestibule SCC, this malignant entity is difficult to diagnose in the early stages, mainly due to its anatomical location and late-stage appearance with vague initial symptoms such as nasal obstruction, chronic nasal secretion, epistaxis, and facial pain [17]. In these anatomical regions, accurately determining the tumor's site of origin can be challenging, particularly in advanced cases. This is particularly true for malignancies involving the maxillary sinus (whether arising from the oral mucosa or sinonasal mucosa), and those affecting both the upper nasal cavities and the nasopharynx (if originating from either site) [18].

Recently, significant attention has turned toward the potential role of the microbiome in influencing the development of head and neck SCC [19]. The human microbiome plays a crucial role in maintaining homeostasis within various body systems; it represents a diverse collection of microorganisms that coexist in symbiotic relationships within various human habitats. It is essential for supporting the immune system and overall health. Because of the unique nature of different microbial niches, the composition of these microorganisms varies in various anatomical sites, such as the airways, digestive system, and skin. The microbiota is affected by various factors, including environmental influences, the age and immune status of the host, and interactions within the microbiota itself. When the balance of the human microbial community is disrupted, beneficial and commensal bacteria that help control the overgrowth of harmful bacteria are often diminished [20].

In the nasal and sinonasal tract, a diverse and balanced microbial community is essential for immune function and mucosal barrier integrity [21]. However, perturbations to this balance, referred to as dysbiosis, have been implicated in various diseases, including allergic rhinitis (AR) and chronic rhinosinusitis (CRS), and now are suspected to contribute to malignancies. Recent evidence indicates that the composition and changes in the microbiome, as well as the presence of specific microbes in certain niches, can initiate tumor formation and promote tumor progression in vivo [22–24]. Furthermore, recent studies have unexpectedly revealed that microbiota play a key role in cancer development, primarily by impacting host cell growth and death, modifying immune system function, and influencing host metabolism [25,26].

Research specifically linking the microbiome to nasal malignancies is still limited. However, the general relationship between microbiota and head and neck cancers suggests that dysbiotic conditions may contribute to carcinogenesis in the nasal district [27]. Some authors reported that inflammation caused by bacterial imbalances might play a role in promoting the development of malignancies in these areas [28]. Further studies are needed to explore this potential connection. The aim of this paper is to review the emerging scientific evidence linking microbial dysbiosis in the nasal vestibule, nasal cavity, and sinonasal district with the development of SCCs. We explore the mechanisms through which an altered microbiome may contribute to carcinogenesis, focusing on chronic inflammation, immune evasion, and pathogen-associated molecular pathways.

We conducted a comprehensive search of all relevant papers across three major medical databases: PubMed, Scopus, and the Cochrane Library. We considered all available documents on the topic from the inception of each database up to September 2024. Additionally, we performed a manual search of the key literature from otolaryngology conferences and used citation chaining to ensure that no relevant articles were overlooked. The search utilized a combination of key terms: "Microbiota", "Microbiome", "Nasal", "Nose vestibule", "Carcinoma", "Cancer", and "Tumor". The inclusion criteria focused on original articles, encompassing both prospective and retrospective studies, as well as review articles. Exclusions were made for single case reports, conference papers, articles not published in English, and letters to the editor.

2. The Nasal Microbiome: An Overview

The nasal district hosts a diverse range of microorganisms, including bacteria, fungi, and viruses. In healthy individuals, the nasal microbiota helps maintain mucosal integrity, modulates immune responses, and protects against colonization by pathogenic organisms. This is important because the upper airway is constantly exposed to airflow from the external environment. As such, the upper airways play essential physiological roles, including humidifying, warming, and filtering inhaled air. The nasal cavities connect to the external environment via the nasal vestibule, acting as a crucial transition zone that links the outside to the lower airways and the gastrointestinal system. Additionally, individuals inhale around 10^4–10^6 biological particles per cubic meter of air daily. Beyond these biological particles, the upper airways are subjected to physical and chemical weathering agents, such as humidity, oxygen, and various immunological or nutritional factors. These factors are significant as they contribute to the development of distinct microenvironments within different regions of the upper airway, including the nasal vestibule, nasal cavities, paranasal sinuses, nasopharynx, Eustachian tubes, middle ear cavities, oral cavity, oropharynx, and larynx. As a result, these different microenvironments in the upper airway host distinct microbial communities composed of both transient and resident microorganisms in differing ratios [29].

In the literature, the most commonly reported sampling sites for analyzing the upper airway microbiome are the nasal vestibule, middle meatus, and nasopharynx. The primary function of the nasal mucosa, which involves clearing inhaled air, may contribute to the high diversity observed in mucosal samples across these areas [30,31].

The nasal vestibule surface, with its epithelium comprising sebaceous glands and vibrissae, is relatively drier compared to other regions of the upper airway and is the most exposed to the external environment. These vibrissae are able to trap larger particles (>3 μm) from inhaled air, while smaller particles, including microorganisms, are captured in a layer of mucus lining the nasal cavity. This mucus is then transported by ciliated epithelial cells from the nose to the esophagus through a process identified as mucociliary clearance [32,33]. The middle meatus is particularly significant for nasal microbiome research because it serves as the convergence point for secretions from the anterior part of the nasal cavity, anterior ethmoid, maxillary sinus, and frontal sinus [34]. The microbial community of the nasal vestibule is primarily dominated by species belonging to the genus *Corynebacterium*, *Staphylococcus*, *Propionibacterium*, and *Moraxella*. Notably, the nasal vestibule serves as a key reservoir for *Staphylococcus aureus* [35]. Regarding the sinonasal tract, this area includes rich diverse bacterial communities, with *Staphylococcus aureus*, *Staphylococcus epidermidis*, and *Propionibacterium acnes* representing the most abundant species [36]. The nasal microbiome usually correlates with the skin microbiome and, due to its lower complexity compared to, for instance, the oral microbiome, it is more susceptible to changes caused by environmental factors that can disrupt this delicate balance [37]. Such distruptions can lead to colonization [38] and proliferation of potentially opportunistic species that, by altering the immune homeostasis, may contribute to chronic inflammatory states, such as AR and CRS [39,40]. In patients with CRS, studies have reported a decrease in microbial diversity and an overrepresentation of certain bacteria, such as *Staphylococcus aureus* and *Pseudomonas aeruginosa* [41]. This imbalance is associated with prolonged inflammation and mucosal damage, which, over time, may increase the risk of developing malignancies [42] as described in Figure 1.

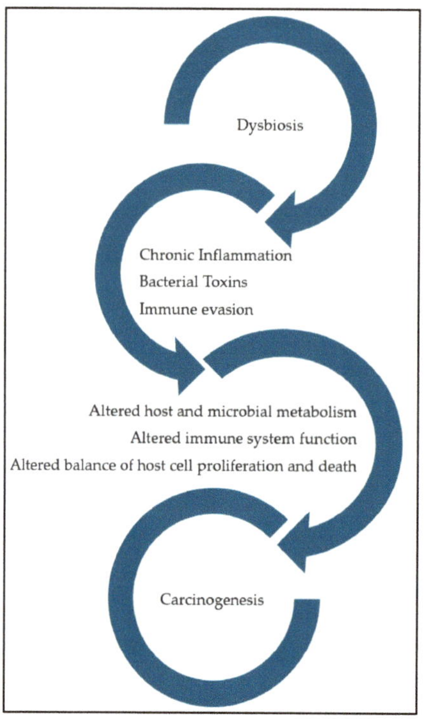

Figure 1. Potential implications of dysbiosis contributing to carcinogenesis.

3. Mechanisms Linking Dysbiosis to Carcinogenesis

3.1. Chronic Inflammation

One of the primary mechanisms through which microbial dysbiosis can potentially contribute to nasal SCC is chronic inflammation [28].

In healthy individuals, the nasal mucosa is constantly exposed to environmental antigens and microorganisms. The nasal microbiome plays an essential role in modulating local immune responses and preventing excessive inflammation. However, colonization and overgrowth of bacteria capable of triggering and sustaining inflammatory responses may impair the local homeostasis, which is otherwise maintained by the nasal microbiome that modulates local immune responses to prevent excessive inflammation. In this regard, Gan et al. emphasized that the recurrence of chronic rhinosinusitis with nasal polyps (CRSwNP) after adequate endoscopic sinus surgery may potentially be associated with a state of dysbiosis, specifically characterized by a decreased presence of protective microorganisms and a higher prevalence of pathogenic microorganisms, including *Staphylococcus aureus* [43].

Chronic inflammation is a well-established risk factor for cancer in various tissues. Several authors report that long-term inflammation leads to the production of reactive oxygen species (ROS) and pro-inflammatory cytokines and chemokines, which can cause DNA damage, disrupt cellular processes, and promote malignant transformation. ROS have long been linked to cancer, with various tumor cells exhibiting elevated ROS levels compared to their normal counterparts. These increased ROS levels are believed to be oncogenic, leading to damage in DNA, proteins, and lipids, which in turn promotes genetic instability and tumorigenesis. Additionally, ROS function as signaling molecules in cancer, contributing to abnormal cell proliferation, metastasis, resistance to apoptosis, and angiogenesis, as well as causing differentiation blocks in certain cancer types. Elevated ROS levels create a pro-tumorigenic environment by activating pro-survival signaling pathways, impairing tumor suppressor gene function, enhancing glucose metabolism, enabling adaptations to hypoxia, and fostering the emergence of oncogenic mutations [44–46]. A further mechanism in bacterial carcinogenesis entails the activation of nuclear factor kappa B (NF-κB), which represents a crucial player in this process. Specifically, NF-κB is activated by several bacterial components, triggering the release of pro-inflammatory cytokines, which are related to cancer development [47]. Likewise, the activation of tumor necrosis factor alpha (TNF-α) and multiple inflammatory cytokines, including IL-6, IL-10, and IL-23, play a critical role in the cancer-promoting mechanisms associated with certain microbes [48].

Additionally, smoking can interfere with the balance of the nasal microbiome and increase the colonization by pathogenic bacteria [49–51]. It is widely acknowledged as a significant contributor to the development of nasal and sinonasal SCC, particularly in the malignant degeneration of sinonasal inverted papilloma [52]. Also, regarding the nasal vestibule, smoking is considered a risk factor for the development of SCC, as various studies in the literature show that the majority of patients with SCC are either smokers or former smokers [53].

Interestingly, Beachler et al. emphasized that chronic sinusitis may play a role in the development of some head and neck cancers, including nasopharyngeal cancer, HPV-related oropharyngeal cancer, and cancers of the nasal cavity and paranasal sinuses, potentially due to immunodeficiency or chronic inflammation [54].

3.2. Immune Evasion

An altered microbiome can significantly impair the local immune response, which may facilitate the persistence of potentially malignant cells within the tissue. In a healthy physiological state, the immune system plays a crucial role in actively surveilling and eliminating any abnormal or pre-cancerous cells that may arise. However, under conditions of dysbiosis, certain bacterial species may become predominant and produce various factors that can suppress immune function or promote mechanisms of immune evasion. This disruption in the balance of microbial communities can, therefore, compromise the immune system's ability to effectively target and eliminate these potentially harmful cells [55]. For instance, *Staphylococcus aureus*, frequently overrepresented in dysbiotic nasal microbiomes, secretes superantigens and other virulence factors that can disrupt normal immune responses [56–58].

3.3. Direct Carcinogenic Effects of Bacterial Toxins

Certain bacterial species have the capacity to produce toxins and metabolites that directly promote carcinogenesis. For instance, chronic inflammation caused by ongoing *Staphylococcus aureus* infections can result in DNA damage, interfere with cellular signaling pathways, and contribute to the creation of an immunosuppressive microenvironment that promotes and supports cancer development. Furthermore, *Staphylococcus aureus* produces various toxins and metabolites that can interact directly with host cells, potentially leading to oncogenic changes. Indeed, chronic *Staphylococcus aureus* infections have been associated with an increased risk of skin cancer and oral cancer [59].

Another bacterium that can colonize the nasal mucosa is *Pseudomonas aeruginosa*, which produces important virulence factors, including pyocyanin, which triggers ROS production, causing oxidative stress in epithelial cells [60]. Over time, this oxidative stress can result in genetic mutations, genomic instability, and cellular transformation, paving the way for malignancy. In this regard, a *Pseudomonas* infection of the nose has been reported in some cases as an unusual complication of nasal surgery, or as an etiological agent of rhinosinusitis in immunocompromised patients [61,62].

A summary of the aforementioned mechanisms linking dysbiosis to carcinogenesis is presented in Table 1.

Table 1. Mechanisms linking dysbiosis to carcinogenesis.

Mechanisms Linking Dysbiosis to Carcinogenesis	Molecular Mediator	Molecular Mechanism	References
Chronic Inflammation	Reactive oxygen species	DNA damage Cellular process disruption Malignant transformation promotion	[44–46]
	Nuclear factor kappa B		[47]
	Tumor necrosis factor α		[48]
	Inflammatory cytokines		
Immune Evasion	Superantigens and other virulence factors secretion (*Staphylococcus aureus*)	Normal immune response disruption	[56–58]
Bacterial Toxins	Toxins and metabolites production (*Staphylococcus aureus*)	DNA damage Interference with cellular signaling Immunosuppressive environment	[59]
	Pyocyanin (*Pseudomonas aeruginosa*)	Reactive oxygen species triggering	[60]

4. Fungal and Viral Contributions to Nasal Carcinogenesis

Fungi and viruses may play a crucial role in nasal carcinogenesis, either independently or through interactions with the bacterial microbiome.

4.1. Fungal Involvement

Fungal communities that inhabit our bodies are collectively known as the mycobiome. This mycobiome is frequently overlooked as a possible factor in disease development, mainly because it is less abundant (<0.1% of the total microbiota) and less diverse. Despite this, fungi are considerably larger than bacteria and possess metabolic gene clusters that align with various ecological requirements. Compared to the bacteriome, information about the mycobiome is limited. However, the recent application of advanced genomic sequencing techniques in fungal studies has enhanced our knowledge of their roles in health and disease. The mycobiome can be located in various anatomical regions including the oral cavity, airways, skin, vagina, and gastrointestinal tract [63].

In contrast to the bacterial microbiome, there has been a lack of studies investigating the sinus mycobiome in nasal inflammatory conditions; the most recent findings about this topic have highlighted that, like the bacterial microbiome, decreased fungal diversity may play a significant role in the mechanism of nasal dysbiosis.

Differences in mycobiome diversity between CRS patients and healthy individuals indicate that changes in the fungal mycobiome may contribute to disease pathogenesis in a manner similar to the bacterial microbiome [64].

Fungi, such as *Aspergillus* and *Candida*, have been implicated in the chronic inflammation associated with sinonasal diseases [65]. Chronic fungal infections that have persisted over long periods can significantly contribute to ongoing mucosal irritation and disrupt normal immune function, thereby creating an environment that may facilitate the development of malignancy.

4.2. *Viral Involvement*

Viruses are responsible for about 10% to 15% of all cancer cases globally. Various viruses have been implicated in the development of cancer, particularly several DNA viruses, which include Kaposi's sarcoma herpesvirus (KSHV), Merkel cell polyomavirus (MCV), Human Papilloma Virus (HPV), Epstein–Barr virus (EBV), Hepatitis B virus (HBV), and Simian virus 40 (SV40). In addition, there are at least two RNA viruses involved in carcinogenesis: Human T-lymphotropic virus-1 (HTLV-1) and Hepatitis C virus (HCV). Notably, HPV and EBV are the oncogenic viruses most commonly linked to cancers of the head and neck region [66].

4.2.1. Human Papilloma Virus (HPV)

The incidence of head and neck cancers related to HPV has been on the rise, as evidenced by the increasing rates of oropharyngeal squamous cell carcinoma (OPSCC) over the past few decades [67]. Recently, research has focused on the virus's role in these cancers, with studies highlighting its prognostic significance in OPSCC [68]. Although HPV plays a clear etiological role in certain head and neck squamous cell carcinomas, the involvement of HPV in nasal malignancies is less clear. Recent studies have suggested that the presence of HPV in the sinonasal cavities, coupled with microbiome dysbiosis, may contribute to malignancy by allowing persistent viral infection [69,70]. Interestingly, it has been reported that up to 25% of malignancies arising in the sinonasal district contain transcriptionally active HPV [71]. Moreover, the virus is supposed to contribute to the transformation of sinonasal inverted papillomas into malignant carcinomas [72,73].

Furthermore, there are some reports in the literature of HPV being involved in the etiopathogenesis of nasal vestibule carcinoma. In this regard, Vital et al. examined p16 overexpression and high-risk human papilloma virus (HR-HPV) infection in nasal vestibule SCC, revealing a correlation between HR-HPV and p16 overexpression but without any influence on the outcome [74]. Yamamura et al. examined the presence of HPV-DNA using polymerase chain reaction (PCR) and assessed p16 status in five patients affected by nasal vestibule SCC. Three of these patients were treated with chemoradiation therapy, one with surgery, and one with surgery followed by radiation therapy. The authors found that four of the five cases were p16-positive, and one case was positive for HR-HPV infection [75]. Owusu-Ayim et al. described a 68-year-old man affected by SCC of the nasal vestibule. Immunohistochemistry revealed that the lesion was characterized by a surface epithelium exhibiting high-grade cytonuclear atypia and was positive for p16 and HPV infection [76].

4.2.2. Epstein–Barr Virus (EBV)

Interestingly Epstein–Barr Virus (EBV) has been found in a significant proportion of sinonasal SCCs [77]. However, since a similar proportion of EBV infection was detected in nasal polyps, its effective role in sinonasal SCC carcinogenesis should be considered questionable [78]. Also, for the nasal vestibule, studies investigating the role of EBV in SCC are rare, and specifically, Paulino et al. found no association between nasal vestibule SCC and Epstein–Barr Virus infection [79].

5. Clinical Implications and Potential Therapeutic Approaches

5.1. *Microbiome-Targeted Interventions*

Probiotic therapies, designed to increase microbial diversity and promote the growth of beneficial commensal bacteria, are currently being explored in other cancers [80]. Further research is needed to understand whether this therapeutic strategy could potentially be applied to nasal malignancies.

Current research demonstrates the effectiveness of probiotics in the potential prevention of cancer and as an adjunctive treatment during anticancer chemotherapy. However, clinical trials remain insufficient to definitively confirm the potential of probiotic microorganisms in this context [81].

Upper respiratory tract probiotics, encompassing both traditional Lactobacillales and next-generation candidate probiotics (e.g., Dolosigranulum), may provide a natural support to standard treatment options. Although this area remains relatively underexplored compared to gut probiotic research, the application of probiotics in topical formulations is noteworthy. They have the potential to address various aspects of upper respiratory tract diseases due to their multifaceted mechanisms of action, which include microbiome restoration, antimicrobial activity, immunomodulation, and enhancement of barrier function [82].

5.2. *Antibiotic and Antifungal Therapies*

In cases where pathogenic bacteria or fungi are detected, targeted antibiotic or antifungal treatments may reduce inflammation and restore normal mucosal function. However, indiscriminate use of antibiotics could further disrupt the microbiome and increase the risk of developing prolonged inflammatory conditions such as CRS, underscoring the need for precision medicine approaches that take individual microbiome profiles into account [83].

5.3. *Immunotherapy*

Since dysbiosis is associated with immune dysfunction, combining microbiome modulation with immunotherapies may be a promising approach for treating nasal SCC in the advanced stage [84]. Enhancing the immune system's ability to detect and eliminate malignant cells, while simultaneously restoring microbial balance, could improve clinical outcomes for patients.

Currently, immune checkpoint inhibitors (ICIs) are recognized as one of the first-line therapies for many unresectable solid tumors. However, evidence regarding the efficacy of ICIs in sinonasal malignancies is limited, and no ICIs have been approved for use in treating sinonasal SCC to date [85].

6. Future Directions for Research

The area of microbiome research specifically related to nasal malignancies is still in its very early stages of development, and a significant amount remains to be thoroughly understood and clarified. Future studies should aim to systematically characterize the microbiome in larger and more diverse cohorts of patients diagnosed with nasal vestibule or sinonasal SCC in order to expand the existing findings; carefully explore the causal relationships that exist between specific microbial species and the complex process of carcinogenesis by utilizing both animal models and in vitro experimental systems; and rigorously investigate the potential for microbiome-based biomarkers to aid in the early detection, diagnosis, and risk stratification for various types of nasal malignancies. Furthermore, additional research is also critically needed to explore the possible role of the mycobiome (the fungal microbiome) and the virome (the viral microbiome) in the intricate context of nasal carcinogenesis.

7. Conclusions

The relationship between microbial dysbiosis and nasal SCCs is an emerging area of scientific inquiry. Alterations in the nasal microbiome, characterized by decreased diversity and the overrepresentation of pathogenic microorganisms, appear to play a significant role in promoting chronic inflammation and immune evasion, and may promote carcinogenesis. While more research is needed to fully elucidate the mechanisms at play, understanding the role of the microbiome in nasal vestibular and non-vestibular SCCs could pave the way for novel therapeutic interventions aimed at preventing these aggressive malignancies.

Author Contributions: Conceptualization, A.L. and B.F.; methodology, A.T. and L.M.; data curation, D.R.; writing and original draft preparation, A.L.; writing, review, and editing, A.L. and B.F.; validation, L.T., G.B., G.D. and F.B. All authors have read and agreed to the published version of the manuscript.

Funding: This research received no external funding.

Data Availability Statement: No new data were created or analyzed in this study. Data sharing is not applicable to this article.

Conflicts of Interest: The authors declare no conflicts of interest.

References

1. Turner, J.H.; Reh, D.D. Incidence and survival in patients with sinonasal cancer: A historical analysis of population-based data. *Head Neck* **2012**, *34*, 877–885. [CrossRef] [PubMed]
2. Dulguerov, P.; Allal, A.S. Nasal and paranasal sinus carcinoma: How can we continue to make progress? *Curr. Opin. Otolaryngol. Head Neck Surg.* **2006**, *14*, 67–72. [CrossRef] [PubMed]
3. Bussu, F.; Tagliaferri, L.; Piras, A.; Rizzo, D.; Tsatsaris, N.; De Corso, E.; Parrilla, C.; Paludetti, G. Multidisciplinary approach to nose vestibule malignancies: Setting new standards. *Acta Otorhinolaryngol. Ital.* **2021**, *41*, 158–165. [CrossRef] [PubMed]
4. Scheurleer, W.F.J.; Tagliaferri, L.; Rijken, J.A.; Crescio, C.; Rizzo, D.; Mattiucci, G.C.; Pameijer, F.A.; de Bree, R.; Fionda, B.; de Ridder, M.; et al. Evaluation of Staging Systems for Cancer of the Nasal Vestibule. *Cancers* **2023**, *15*, 3028. [CrossRef]
5. Scheurleer, W.F.J.; de Ridder, M.; Tagliaferri, L.; Crescio, C.; Parrilla, C.; Mattiucci, G.C.; Fionda, B.; Deganello, A.; Galli, J.; de Bree, R.; et al. Validation of the "Rome" Classification for Squamous Cell Carcinoma of the Nasal Vestibule. *Cancers* **2023**, *16*, 37. [CrossRef] [PubMed]
6. Bussu, F.; Gallus, R.; Rizzo, D.; Tramaloni, P.; Tsatsaris, N.; Tagliaferri, L.; Galli, J.; Nicolai, P. A Proposal for a Consistent Classification of Nasal Vestibule Carcinomas. In *Malignancies of the Nasal Vestibule*; Bussu, F., Ed.; Springer: Cham, Switzerland, 2023. [CrossRef]
7. Bussu, F.; Rizzo, D.; Tramaloni, P.; Rigante, M.; Tsatsaris, N.; Ralli, M.; Gallus, R.; Presutti, L. Peculiar Patterns of Spread of Nose Vestibule Malignancies. In *Malignancies of the Nasal Vestibule*; Bussu, F., Ed.; Springer: Cham, Switzerland, 2023. [CrossRef]
8. Bussu, F.; Tagliaferri, L.; Crescio, C.; Rizzo, D.; Gallus, R.; Parrilla, C.; Fionda, B.; Lancellotta, V.; Mattiucci, G.C.; Galli, J. New standards for the management of nose vestibule malignancies. *Acta Otolaryngol.* **2023**, *143*, 215–222. [CrossRef]
9. Bussu, F.; Tagliaferri, L.; Corbisiero, M.F.; Lotto, C.; Pellini, R.; Guarino, P.; Mercante, G.; Galuppi, A.; Cariti, F.; Almadori, G.; et al. Management of nasal vestibule carcinomas: Recommendations by the Oncological Committee of the Italian Society of Otorhinolaryngology—Head and Neck Surgery. *Acta Otorhinolaryngol.* **2024**, *44*, 13–20. [CrossRef]
10. Testa, G.; Mattavelli, D.; Rampinelli, V.; Conti, C.; Piazza, C. Squamous cell carcinoma of the nasal vestibule: A diagnostic and therapeutic challenge. *Eur. Arch. Otorhinolaryngol.* **2024**, *281*, 5627–5640. [CrossRef]
11. Ferrari, M.; Taboni, S.; Carobbio, A.L.C.; Emanuelli, E.; Maroldi, R.; Bossi, P.; Nicolai, P. Sinonasal Squamous Cell Carcinoma, a Narrative Reappraisal of the Current Evidence. *Cancers* **2021**, *13*, 2835. [CrossRef]
12. Elgart, K.; Faden, D.L. Sinonasal Squamous Cell Carcinoma: Etiology, Pathogenesis, and the Role of Human Papilloma Virus. *Curr. Otorhinolaryngol. Rep.* **2020**, *8*, 111–119. [CrossRef]
13. Binazzi, A.; Ferrante, P.; Marinaccio, A. Occupational exposure and sinonasal cancer: A systematic review and meta-analysis. *BMC Cancer* **2015**, *15*, 49. [CrossRef] [PubMed]
14. Bracigliano, A.; Tatangelo, F.; Perri, F.; Di Lorenzo, G.; Tafuto, R.; Ottaiano, A.; Clemente, O.; Barretta, M.L.; Losito, N.S.; Santorsola, M.; et al. Malignant Sinonasal Tumors: Update on Histological and Clinical Management. *Curr. Oncol.* **2021**, *28*, 2420–2438. [CrossRef]
15. Chang Sing Pang, K.J.W.; Mur, T.; Collins, L.; Rao, S.R.; Faden, D.L. Human Papillomavirus in Sinonasal Squamous Cell Carcinoma: A Systematic Review and Meta-Analysis. *Cancers* **2020**, *13*, 45. [CrossRef]
16. Sbrana, M.F.; Borges, R.F.R.; Pinna, F.R.; Neto, D.B.; Voegels, R.L. Sinonasal inverted papilloma: Rate of recurrence and malignant transformation in 44 operated patients. *Braz. J. Otorhinolaryngol.* **2021**, *87*, 80–84. [CrossRef]

17. Pecorari, G.; Motatto, G.M.; Piazza, F.; Garzaro, A.; Riva, G. Real-Life Prognosis of Sinonasal Tumors. *J. Pers. Med.* **2024**, *14*, 444. [CrossRef] [PubMed]
18. Binazzi, A.; di Marzio, D.; Mensi, C.; Consonni, D.; Miligi, L.; Piro, S.; Zajacovà, J.; Sorasio, D.; Galli, P.; Camagni, A.; et al. Gender Differences in Sinonasal Cancer Incidence: Data from the Italian Registry. *Cancers* **2024**, *16*, 2053. [CrossRef] [PubMed]
19. Sahin, T.K.; Sonmezer, M.C. The role of the microbiome in head and neck squamous cell cancers. *Eur. Arch. Otorhinolaryngol.* **2024**. [CrossRef]
20. Thomas, S.; Izard, J.; Walsh, E.; Batich, K.; Chongsathidkiet, P.; Clarke, G.; Sela, D.A.; Muller, A.J.; Mullin, J.M.; Albert, K.; et al. The Host Microbiome Regulates and Maintains Human Health: A Primer and Perspective for Non-Microbiologists. *Cancer Res.* **2017**, *77*, 1783–1812. [CrossRef]
21. Tai, J.; Han, M.S.; Kwak, J.; Kim, T.H. Association Between Microbiota and Nasal Mucosal Diseases in terms of Immunity. *Int. J. Mol. Sci.* **2021**, *22*, 4744. [CrossRef]
22. Loperfido, A.; Cavaliere, C.; Begvarfaj, E.; Ciofalo, A.; D'Erme, G.; De Vincentiis, M.; Greco, A.; Millarelli, S.; Bellocchi, G.; Masieri, S. The Impact of Antibiotics and Steroids on the Nasal Microbiome in Patients with Chronic Rhinosinusitis: A Systematic Review According to PICO Criteria. *J. Pers. Med.* **2023**, *13*, 1583. [CrossRef]
23. Hwang, S.; Yi, H.C.; Hwang, S.; Jo, M.; Rhee, K.J. Dietary Salt Administration Decreases Enterotoxigenic Bacteroides fragilis (ETBF)-Promoted Tumorigenesis via Inhibition of Colonic Inflammation. *Int. J. Mol. Sci.* **2020**, *21*, 8034. [CrossRef] [PubMed]
24. Parida, S.; Wu, S.; Siddharth, S.; Wang, G.; Muniraj, N.; Nagalingam, A.; Hum, C.; Mistriotis, P.; Hao, H.; Talbot, C.C., Jr.; et al. A Procarcinogenic Colon Microbe Promotes Breast Tumorigenesis and Metastatic Progression and Concomitantly Activates Notch and β-Catenin Axes. *Cancer Discov.* **2021**, *11*, 1138–1157. [CrossRef] [PubMed]
25. Hou, K.; Wu, Z.X.; Chen, X.Y.; Wang, J.Q.; Zhang, D.; Xiao, C.; Zhu, D.; Koya, J.B.; Wei, L.; Li, J.; et al. Microbiota in health and diseases. *Signal Transduct. Target. Ther.* **2022**, *7*, 135. [CrossRef] [PubMed]
26. Wang, Y.; Wang, Y.; Wang, J. A comprehensive analysis of intratumor microbiome in head and neck squamous cell carcinoma. *Eur. Arch. Otorhinolaryngol.* **2022**, *279*, 4127–4136. [CrossRef]
27. Picardo, S.L.; Coburn, B.; Hansen, A.R. The microbiome and cancer for clinicians. *Crit. Rev. Oncol. Hematol.* **2019**, *141*, 1–12. [CrossRef] [PubMed]
28. Wu, E.L.; Riley, C.A.; Hsieh, M.C.; Marino, M.J.; Wu, X.C.; McCoul, E.D. Chronic sinonasal tract inflammation as a precursor to nasopharyngeal carcinoma and sinonasal malignancy in the United States. *Int. Forum Allergy Rhinol.* **2017**, *7*, 786–793. [CrossRef]
29. Di Stadio, A.; Costantini, C.; Renga, G.; Pariano, M.; Ricci, G.; Romani, L. The Microbiota/Host Immune System Interaction in the Nose to Protect from COVID-19. *Life* **2020**, *10*, 345. [CrossRef]
30. Stearns, J.C.; Davidson, C.J.; McKeon, S.; Whelan, F.J.; Fontes, M.E.; Schryvers, A.B.; Bowdish, D.M.; Kellner, J.D.; Surette, M.G. Culture and molecular-based profiles show shifts in bacterial communities of the upper respiratory tract that occur with age. *ISME J.* **2015**, *9*, 1246–1259. [CrossRef]
31. Luna, P.N.; Hasegawa, K.; Ajami, N.J.; Espinola, J.A.; Henke, D.M.; Petrosino, J.F.; Piedra, P.A.; Sullivan, A.F.; Camargo, C.A., Jr.; Shaw, C.A.; et al. The association between anterior nares and nasopharyngeal microbiota in infants hospitalized for bronchiolitis. *Microbiome* **2018**, *6*, 2. [CrossRef]
32. Cohen, N.A. Sinonasal mucociliary clearance in health and disease. *Ann. Otol. Rhinol. Laryngol. Suppl.* **2006**, *196*, 20–26. [CrossRef]
33. Yan, M.; Pamp, S.J.; Fukuyama, J.; Hwang, P.H.; Cho, D.Y.; Holmes, S.; Relman, D.A. Nasal microenvironments and interspecific interactions influence nasal microbiota complexity and S. aureus carriage. *Cell Host Microbe* **2013**, *14*, 631–640. [CrossRef] [PubMed]
34. Reddy, U.D.; Dev, B. Pictorial essay: Anatomical variations of paranasal sinuses on multidetector computed tomography-How does it help FESS surgeons? *Indian J. Radiol. Imaging* **2012**, *22*, 317–324. [CrossRef]
35. Kluytmans, J.A.; Wertheim, H.F. Nasal carriage of Staphylococcus aureus and prevention of nosocomial infections. *Infection* **2005**, *33*, 3–8. [CrossRef]
36. Rawls, M.; Ellis, A.K. The microbiome of the nose. *Ann. Allergy Asthma Immunol.* **2019**, *122*, 17–24. [CrossRef]
37. Zhou, X.; Shen, X.; Johnson, J.S.; Spakowicz, D.J.; Agnello, M.; Zhou, W.; Avina, M.; Honkala, A.; Chleilat, F.; Chen, S.J.; et al. Longitudinal profiling of the microbiome at four body sites reveals core stability and individualized dynamics during health and disease. *Cell Host Microbe* **2024**, *32*, 506–526. [CrossRef] [PubMed]
38. Belkaid, Y.; Hand, T.W. Role of the microbiota in immunity and inflammation. *Cell* **2014**, *157*, 121–141. [CrossRef]
39. Capponi, M.; Gori, A.; De Castro, G.; Ciprandi, G.; Anania, C.; Brindisi, G.; Tosca, M.; Cinicola, B.L.; Salvatori, A.; Loffredo, L.; et al. (R)Evolution in Allergic Rhinitis Add-On Therapy: From Probiotics to Postbiotics and Parabiotics. *J. Clin. Med.* **2022**, *11*, 5154. [CrossRef] [PubMed]
40. Huntley, K.S.; Raber, J.; Fine, L.; Bernstein, J.A. Influence of the Microbiome on Chronic Rhinosinusitis With and Without Polyps: An Evolving Discussion. *Front. Allergy* **2021**, *2*, 737086. [CrossRef]
41. Cope, E.K.; Goldberg, A.N.; Pletcher, S.D.; Lynch, S.V. Compositionally and functionally distinct sinus microbiota in chronic rhinosinusitis patients have immunological and clinically divergent consequences. *Microbiome* **2017**, *5*, 53. [CrossRef]
42. Garrett, W.S. Cancer and the microbiota. *Science* **2015**, *348*, 80–86. [CrossRef]
43. Gan, W.; Zhang, H.; Yang, F.; Liu, S.; Liu, F.; Meng, J. The influence of nasal microbiome diversity and inflammatory patterns on the prognosis of nasal polyps. *Sci. Rep.* **2021**, *11*, 6364. [CrossRef] [PubMed]

44. Yu, W.; Tu, Y.; Long, Z.; Liu, J.; Kong, D.; Peng, J.; Wu, H.; Zheng, G.; Zhao, J.; Chen, Y.; et al. Reactive Oxygen Species Bridge the Gap between Chronic Inflammation and Tumor Development. *Oxid. Med. Cell. Longev.* **2022**, *2022*, 2606928. [CrossRef] [PubMed]
45. Moloney, J.N.; Cotter, T.G. ROS signalling in the biology of cancer. *Semin. Cell Dev. Biol.* **2018**, *80*, 50–64. [CrossRef] [PubMed]
46. Renaudin, X. Reactive oxygen species and DNA damage response in cancer. *Int. Rev. Cell Mol. Biol.* **2021**, *364*, 139–161. [CrossRef]
47. Zhang, T.; Ma, C.; Zhang, Z.; Zhang, H.; Hu, H. NF-κB signaling in inflammation and cancer. *MedComm* **2021**, *2*, 618–653. [CrossRef]
48. Heo, G.; Lee, Y.; Im, E. Interplay between the Gut Microbiota and Inflammatory Mediators in the Development of Colorectal Cancer. *Cancers* **2021**, *13*, 734. [CrossRef]
49. Pfeiffer, S.; Herzmann, C.; Gaede, K.I.; Kovacevic, D.; Krauss-Etschmann, S.; Schloter, M. Different responses of the oral, nasal and lung microbiomes to cigarette smoke. *Thorax* **2022**, *77*, 191–195. [CrossRef]
50. Ramakrishnan, V.R.; Frank, D.N. Impact of cigarette smoking on the middle meatus microbiome in health and chronic rhinosinusitis. *Int. Forum Allergy Rhinol.* **2015**, *5*, 981–989. [CrossRef] [PubMed]
51. Uhliarova, B.; Adamkov, M.; Svec, M.; Calkovska, A. The effect of smoking on CT score, bacterial colonization and distribution of inflammatory cells in the upper airways of patients with chronic rhinosinusitis. *Inhal. Toxicol.* **2014**, *26*, 419–425. [CrossRef]
52. Hong, S.L.; Kim, B.H.; Lee, J.H.; Cho, K.S.; Roh, H.J. Smoking and malignancy in sinonasal inverted papilloma. *Laryngoscope* **2013**, *123*, 1087–1091. [CrossRef]
53. Agger, A.; von Buchwald, C.; Madsen, A.R.; Yde, J.; Lesnikova, I.; Christensen, C.B.; Foghsgaard, S.; Christensen, T.B.; Hansen, H.S.; Larsen, S.; et al. Squamous cell carcinoma of the nasal vestibule 1993–2002: A nationwide retrospective study from DAHANCA. *Head Neck* **2009**, *31*, 1593–1599. [CrossRef] [PubMed]
54. Beachler, D.C.; Engels, E.A. Chronic Sinusitis and Risk of Head and Neck Cancer in the US Elderly Population. *JAMA Otolaryngol. Head Neck Surg.* **2017**, *143*, 25–31. [CrossRef] [PubMed]
55. Pickard, J.M.; Zeng, M.Y.; Caruso, R.; Núñez, G. Gut microbiota: Role in pathogen colonization, immune responses, and inflammatory disease. *Immunol. Rev.* **2017**, *279*, 70–89. [CrossRef] [PubMed]
56. Lee, S.; Lane, A.P. Chronic rhinosinusitis as a multifactorial inflammatory disorder. *Curr. Infect. Dis. Rep.* **2011**, *13*, 159–168. [CrossRef]
57. Ramakrishnan, V.R.; Hauser, L.J.; Frank, D.N. The sinonasal bacterial microbiome in health and disease. *Curr. Opin. Otolaryngol. Head Neck Surg.* **2016**, *24*, 20–25. [CrossRef]
58. Vickery, T.W.; Ramakrishnan, V.R.; Suh, J.D. The Role of Staphylococcus aureus in Patients with Chronic Sinusitis and Nasal Polyposis. *Curr. Allergy Asthma Rep.* **2019**, *19*, 21. [CrossRef]
59. Odunitan, T.T.; Apanisile, B.T.; Akinboade, M.W.; Abdulazeez, W.O.; Oyaronbi, A.O.; Ajayi, T.M.; Oyekola, S.A.; Ibrahim, N.O.; Nafiu, T.; Afolabi, H.O.; et al. Microbial mysteries: Staphylococcus aureus and the enigma of carcinogenesis. *Microb. Pathog.* **2024**, *194*, 106831. [CrossRef] [PubMed]
60. Gudis, D.; Zhao, K.Q.; Cohen, N.A. Acquired cilia dysfunction in chronic rhinosinusitis. *Am. J. Rhinol. Allergy* **2012**, *26*, 1–6. [CrossRef]
61. Demir, C.I.; Yaşar, E.K.; Alagöz, M.Ş. Synchronous Pseudomonas Infection in Nose and Maxillery Sinus After Septorhinoplasty. *J. Craniofacial Surg.* **2022**, *33*, 578–580. [CrossRef]
62. Fried, M.P.; Kelly, J.H.; Strome, M. Pseudomonas rhinosinusitis. *Laryngoscope* **1984**, *94*, 192–196. [CrossRef]
63. Gamal, A.; Elshaer, M.; Alabdely, M.; Kadry, A.; McCormick, T.S.; Ghannoum, M. The Mycobiome: Cancer Pathogenesis, Diagnosis, and Therapy. *Cancers* **2022**, *14*, 2875. [CrossRef] [PubMed]
64. Lee, J.T.; Simpson, C.A.; Yang, H.H.; Suh, J.D.; Wang, M.B.; Lagishetty, V.; Liang, F.; Jacobs, J.P. Fungal and Bacterial Microbiome in Sinus Mucosa of Patients with and without Chronic Rhinosinusitis. *Laryngoscope* **2024**, *134*, 1054–1062. [CrossRef] [PubMed]
65. Swarajyalakshmi, M.; Jyothilakshmi, G. Candida kefyr in Invasive Paranasal Sinusitis. *Indian. J. Otolaryngol. Head Neck Surg.* **2014**, *66*, 371–374. [CrossRef]
66. Chen, Y.; Williams, V.; Filippova, M.; Filippov, V.; Duerksen-Hughes, P. Viral carcinogenesis: Factors inducing DNA damage and virus integration. *Cancers* **2014**, *6*, 2155–2186. [CrossRef] [PubMed]
67. Hartwig, S.; Syrjänen, S.; Dominiak-Felden, G.; Brotons, M.; Castellsagué, X. Estimation of the epidemiological burden of human papillomavirus-related cancers and non-malignant diseases in men in Europe: A review. *BMC Cancer* **2012**, *12*, 30. [CrossRef]
68. Lewis, A.; Kang, R.; Levine, A.; Maghami, E. The New Face of Head and Neck Cancer: The HPV Epidemic. *Oncology* **2015**, *29*, 616–626.
69. Lewis, J.S., Jr.; Westra, W.H.; Thompson, L.D.; Barnes, L.; Cardesa, A.; Hunt, J.L.; Williams, M.D.; Slootweg, P.J.; Triantafyllou, A.; Woolgar, J.A.; et al. The sinonasal tract: Another potential "hot spot" for carcinomas with transcriptionally-active human papillomavirus. *Head Neck Pathol.* **2014**, *8*, 241–249. [CrossRef]
70. Hebsgaard, M.; Eriksen, P.; Ramberg, I.; von Buchwald, C. Human Papillomavirus in Sinonasal Malignancies. *Curr. Otorhinolaryngol. Rep.* **2023**, *11*, 109–116. [CrossRef]
71. Bishop, J.A.; Guo, T.W.; Smith, D.F.; Wang, H.; Ogawa, T.; Pai, S.I.; Westra, W.H. Human papillomavirus-related carcinomas of the sinonasal tract. *Am. J. Surg. Pathol.* **2013**, *37*, 185–192. [CrossRef]
72. Kılıç, S.; Kılıç, S.S.; Kim, E.S.; Baredes, S.; Mahmoud, O.; Gray, S.T.; Eloy, J.A. Significance of human papillomavirus positivity in sinonasal squamous cell carcinoma. *Int. Forum Allergy Rhinol.* **2017**, *7*, 980–989. [CrossRef]

73. But-Hadzic, J.; Jenko, K.; Poljak, M.; Kocjan, B.J.; Gale, N.; Strojan, P. Sinonasal inverted papilloma associated with squamous cell carcinoma. *Radiol. Oncol.* **2011**, *45*, 267–272. [CrossRef] [PubMed]
74. Vital, D.; Holzmann, D.; Huber, G.F.; Soyka, M.B.; Moch, H.; Zimmermann, D.R.; Ikenberg, K. p16INK4a: A surrogate marker of high-risk human papillomavirus infection in squamous cell carcinoma of the nasal vestibule. *Head Neck* **2017**, *39*, 1392–1398. [CrossRef] [PubMed]
75. Yamamura, K.; Saito, Y.; Kobayashi, K.; Mukai, T.; Fukuoka, O.; Akashi, K.; Yoshida, M.; Ando, M.; Yamasoba, T. p16 status and high-risk human papilloma virus infection in squamous cell carcinoma of the nasal vestibule. *Auris Nasus Larynx* **2023**, *50*, 942–947. [CrossRef] [PubMed]
76. Owusu-Ayim, M.; Shahsavari, S.; Manickavasagam, J. A Case of Human Papillomavirus-positive Nasal Vestibule Squamous Cell Carcinoma. *Int. J. Head Neck Surg.* **2023**, *14*, 36–39. [CrossRef]
77. Doescher, J.; Piontek, G.; Wirth, M.; Bettstetter, M.; Schlegel, J.; Haller, B.; Brockhoff, G.; Reiter, R.; Pickhard, A. Epstein-Barr virus infection is strictly associated with the metastatic spread of sinonasal squamous-cell carcinomas. *Oral Oncol.* **2015**, *51*, 929–934. [CrossRef]
78. Nukpook, T.; Ekalaksananan, T.; Teeramatwanich, W.; Patarapadungkit, N.; Chaiwiriyakul, S.; Vatanasapt, P.; Aromseree, S.; Pientong, C. Prevalence and association of Epstein-Barr virus infection with sinonasal inverted papilloma and sinonasal squamous cell carcinoma in the northeastern Thai population. *Infect. Agents Cancer* **2020**, *15*, 43. [CrossRef]
79. Paulino, A.F.; Singh, B.; Carew, J.; Shah, J.P.; Huvos, A.G. Epstein-Barr virus in squamous carcinoma of the anterior nasal cavity. *Ann. Diagn. Pathol.* **2000**, *4*, 7–10. [CrossRef]
80. Bhatt, A.P.; Redinbo, M.R.; Bultman, S.J. The role of the microbiome in cancer development and therapy. *CA Cancer J. Clin.* **2017**, *67*, 326–344. [CrossRef]
81. Śliżewska, K.; Markowiak-Kopeć, P.; Śliżewska, W. The Role of Probiotics in Cancer Prevention. *Cancers* **2020**, *13*, 20. [CrossRef]
82. De Boeck, I.; Spacova, I.; Vanderveken, O.M.; Lebeer, S. Lactic acid bacteria as probiotics for the nose? *Microb. Biotechnol.* **2021**, *14*, 859–869. [CrossRef]
83. Maxfield, A.Z.; Korkmaz, H.; Gregorio, L.L.; Busaba, N.Y.; Gray, S.T.; Holbrook, E.H.; Guo, R.; Bleier, B.S. General antibiotic exposure is associated with increased risk of developing chronic rhinosinusitis. *Laryngoscope* **2017**, *127*, 296–302. [CrossRef] [PubMed]
84. Kuo, Y.H.; Lin, C.S. Regression of advanced maxillary sinus cancer with orbital invasion by combined chemotherapy and immunotherapy: A one-year follow-up case report. *Mol. Clin. Oncol.* **2022**, *16*, 94. [CrossRef] [PubMed]
85. Chen, F.; Zhang, H.; Li, Y.; Liang, T.; Zhang, T. Complete remission in a patient with sinonasal squamous cell carcinoma receiving neoadjuvant tislelizumab plus chemotherapy: A case report. *Front. Immunol.* **2024**, *15*, 1414529. [CrossRef] [PubMed]

medicina

MDPI

Article

Underlying Diagnosis of Food Bolus Obstruction Acute Admissions to Otorhinolaryngology: A Shift to Provide the Best Care as per the Current Guidelines

Rasads Misirovs [1,2,*], Anna Kamusella [3], Michael Miller [4] and Samit Majumdar [5]

1 Department of Otorhinolaryngology, NHS Lothian, Edinburgh EH16 4SA, UK
2 Department of Doctoral Studies, Riga Stradins University, LV-1007 Riga, Latvia
3 Department of Psychiatry, Edinburgh, NHS Lothian, Edinburgh EH10 5HF, UK
4 Department of Gastroenterology, Ninewells Hospital & Medical School, NHS Tayside, Dundee DD1 9SY, UK
5 Department of Otorhinolaryngology, Ninewells Hospital & Medical School, NHS Tayside, Dundee DD1 9SY, UK
* Correspondence: rasads.misirovs@nhs.scot

Abstract: *Background and Objectives:* In the United Kingdom, some patients with food bolus obstruction (FBO) are admitted under the care of ear, nose, and throat (ENT) doctors. In the literature, eosinophilic oesophagitis (EoE) is the most common cause of FBO. We analysed ENT FBO admissions and interventions used in our hospital to investigate for EoE. *Materials and Methods:* This paper details a retrospective study of adult FBO admissions to an ENT ward from January 2016 to December 2019 at a single centre. *Results:* In total, 120 patients were admitted. Half of the patients required instrumentation to resolve the obstruction—31% underwent rigid oesophagoscopy (RO) and 69% oesophagogastroduodenoscopy (OGD). Biopsies were taken during 48% of inpatient OGDs and 5% of ROs. 48% had a histopathological diagnosis of EoE. There was no mention of a specific number of eosinophils per high-power field in 53% of EoE pathology reports. Potentially, some patients were EoE-negative due to an inadequate number of biopsies taken—71% of patients had an insufficient number of biopsies to exclude EoE. A total of 56% of all patients with FBO did not undergo inpatient or outpatient OGDs with biopsies. *Conclusions:* Biopsies were not taken in all FBO patients undergoing oesophagoscopy, leaving EoE underdiagnosed. Follow-up arrangements were often suboptimal to exclude EoE.

Keywords: oesophagogastroduodenoscopy; dysphagia; swallowing disorder; eosinophilic esophagitis; biopsy

1. Introduction

Food, as well as any other material, ingested wilfully or accidentally, can become stuck in the oesophagus, resulting in oesophageal obstruction [1]. Oesophageal food bolus obstruction (FBO) is a common problem, with an estimated annual incidence of 13/100,000 people [2]. Many such cases of obstructions resolve spontaneously. Others may present acutely to hospital emergency departments and subsequently be referred to ear, nose, and throat (ENT) surgeons or gastroenterologists (GIs) for further management [1]. In our health board, patients with soft FBO are admitted to ENT if the suspected obstruction is above the sternal notch; if below the sternal notch, they are admitted under GIs/medics or general surgeons. Ntuli et al. reported that at our institution, between 2008 and 2014, 46.8% of 310 acute FBO admissions were managed by ENT, 43.5% by general surgery, and 9.7% by general medicine [3]. The practice varies between centres in the United Kingdom (UK) depending on a few factors: (1) whether ENT or GI doctors/surgeons

https://doi.org/10.3390/medicina61061047

are in the same hospital with accident and emergency departments, (2) access to flexible oesophagogastroduodenoscopy (OGD) performed by GI doctors or upper GI surgeons in-hours and out-of-hours, and (3) arrangements between ENT, GI doctors, and upper GI surgeons regarding which team patients with FBO are admitted under.

Soft FBO may resolve with 'conservative' strategies. Oesophagoscopy is considered the definitive management for persistent cases of food bolus impaction [1]. The European Society of Gastrointestinal Endoscopy (ESGE) and American Society for Gastrointestinal Endoscopy (ASGEE) recommend definitive management of oesophageal FBO within 24 h to prevent complications from delayed endoscopic interventions. However, the ESGE recommends curative intervention in the first 6 h for complete oesophageal obstruction [1,2]. The inability to swallow one's own saliva and any liquids is suspicious for complete oesophageal obstruction [2].

The advised method of intervention to retrieve a food bolus by the ESGE and the ASGE is flexible endoscopy (primarily OGD, but transnasal oesophagoscopy (TNO) can be used as well), but the ASGE does acknowledge the potential usefulness of rigid oesophagoscopy in higher foreign bodies impacted at the hypopharynx or cricothyroid [4]. The use of flexible or rigid endoscopes carries potentially serious complications [1].

A diagnostic work-up after the removal of the food bolus is recommended to detect any underlying disease, as a lack of appropriate follow-up has been shown to be a predictor for recurrent FBO [2]. The most common predisposing pathology of FBO is eosinophilic oesophagitis (EoE) [3,5]. It is important to take an appropriate number of biopsies from several levels of the oesophagus to diagnose or exclude EoE. Several papers have suggested taking six or more biopsies from three levels of the oesophagus [6]. Biopsy reports are critical diagnostic criteria for EoE, specifically the number of eosinophils per high-power field (hpf). EoE is likely if the eosinophil count per hpf is above 15 hpf [5].

We analysed all admissions for acute FBO to our unit and assessed the type of interventions used and the ability of our processes to diagnose or exclude EoE as the cause of FBO. As EoE is the most common cause of FBO, we intended to see whether appropriate inpatient or outpatient biopsies of the oesophagus were performed to diagnose or exclude EoE. Our study highlights the gap between the current practice and the European guidelines on investigating EoE as the most common cause of FBO [6]. We focused only on ENT-managed FBO, not on GI-managed FBO, as we wanted to assess whether we ENT surgeons investigate our FBO patients well enough according to European guidelines on a condition we deal with rarely in the outpatient setting.

2. Materials and Methods

2.1. Study Design

The STROBE checklist was followed for reporting the findings of this study. This is a retrospective study of adult ($\geq$16 years of age) FBO admissions to the ENT Department in Ninewells Hospital in Dundee, NHS Tayside, Scotland, between January 2016 and December 2019. Patients with FBO were identified through the ENT inpatient ward admission diary. If the same patient had more than one admission during the study period, only the index admission was included in the data analysis. Electronic and paper case notes were accessed. Appropriate clinical governance approvals were granted. Cases of only soft FBO admissions were included in the study; therefore, patients with sharp food objects, such as fishbone or chicken bone, and non-organic foreign bodies were excluded. No standard local protocols were in place specifically, other than already available European guidelines on diagnosing and managing EoE [6].

2.2. Limitations

All NHS Tayside acute admissions with FBO are admitted to Ninewells Hospital. Patients living in the northern part of the NHS Fife area are acutely admitted to Ninewells Hospital, but most of the time, outpatient management of these patients is carried out in Victoria Hospital in Kirkcaldy, NHS Fife; therefore, information on outpatient follow-ups of these patients is not available to NHS Tayside staff. We suspect some of this information on further acute FBO admissions and/or outpatient follow-ups of NHS Fife patients has not been available for our study. Some patients moved outside of the NHS Tayside area since acute admission with FBO to Ninewells Hospital. Overall, we do not have complete follow-up information on 20 such patients.

3. Results

3.1. Demographics

A total of 120 FBO admissions was identified: 82 (68%) were males and 38 (32%) were females. The median age of males was 54.5 (range 16–94) years, while that of females was 69.5 (range 16–92) years, which was statistically significant ($p = 0.008$).

In 87%, the type of food bolus was animal-based, in 8%, it was plant-based, and in the remaining 5%, animal-based food could not be excluded. Of all animal-based food boluses, chicken was the cause of FBO in 36% of admissions, steak—22%, beef—14%, pork—6%, and lamb—5%. The rest was fish, duck, processed food, such as sausages, mince, meatballs, and ham, and unspecified meat; each of these aforementioned food groups was the cause of FBO in less than 5%.

A trend of more admissions during the summer season and winter festive period was noted (Figure 1).

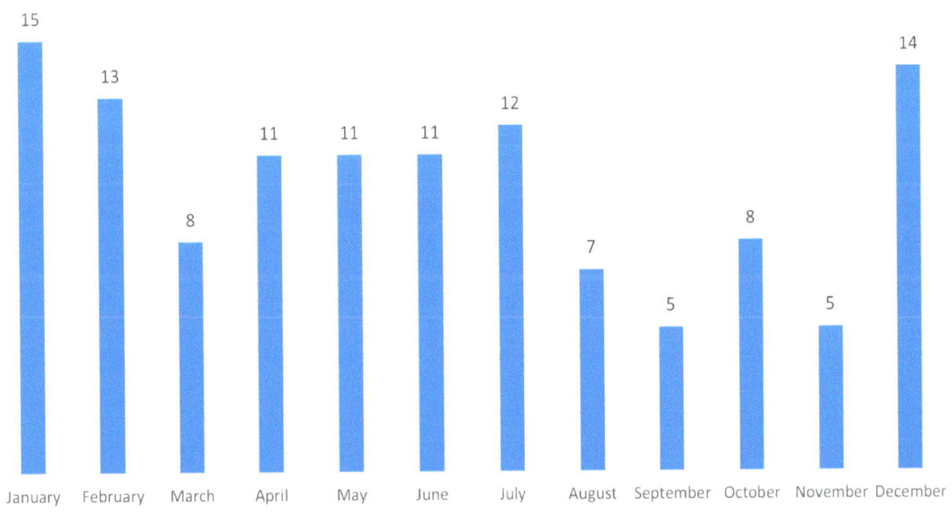

Figure 1. A number of admissions of patients with food bolus obstruction each month of a year.

Several elderly patients were admitted around the time of their birthdays. Admissions during the days of the week were more common on weekends and Mondays (Figure 2).

None of the patients had airway compromise.

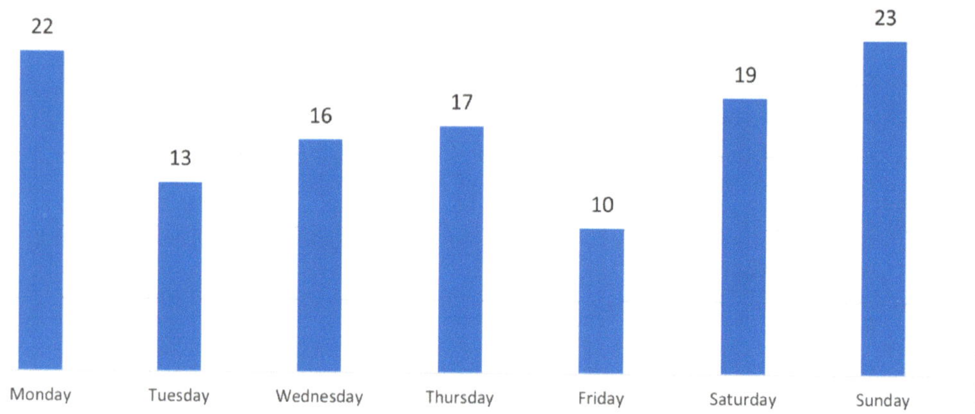

Figure 2. A number of admissions of patients with food bolus obstruction each day of a week.

3.2. *Interventions*

Interestingly, in nearly half (49% or 59/120) of FBO admissions, the obstruction resolved spontaneously within the 24 h observation period. A total of 51% (61/120) of admissions required intervention, rigid oesophagoscopy (RO) or OGD. In 67% (41/61), OGD was the intervention, and in 31% (19/61), it was RO. In one FBO, combined OGD and RO were performed due to cervical osteophytes preventing safe instrumentation with RO.

Two complications of oesophageal tear were recorded, one in the OGD and one in the RO group, leading to a 2.4% and 5.3% complication rate in each group, respectively.

During inpatient OGD, biopsies were taken in 48% (20/42) of cases, while during RO, biopsies were taken in 5% (1/19). Biopsies of inpatient OGD revealed EoE in 50% (10/20) (Figure 3).

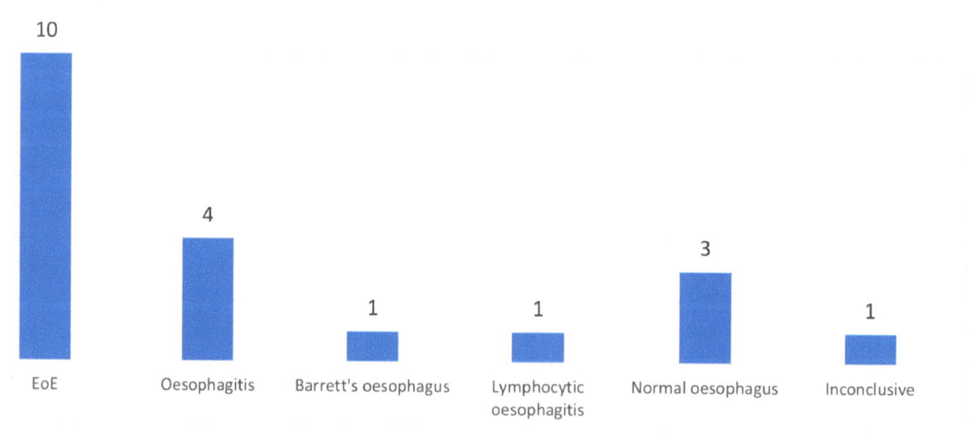

Figure 3. A number of patients with a diagnosis of inpatient OGD biopsies. EoE—eosinophilic oesophagitis.

None of the patients had a previously known diagnosis of EoE.

3.3. Follow-Up

A total of 54% (54/100) of patients in which FBO resolved spontaneously or did not undergo OGD with biopsies during inpatient stay had no follow-up arranged. Outpatient OGD was planned in 16% (16/100) but did not take place in four of the patients for unknown reasons. TNO was planned in 4% (4/100) but did not take place in two of the patients for unknown reasons. An outpatient barium swallow was arranged in 11% (11/100). An outpatient ENT clinic review without OGD/TNO was arranged for 5% (5/100) patients. In 4% (4/100) of the patients, general practitioners (GPs) were advised to request outpatient OGD or barium swallows.

In 92% of outpatient OGDs (11/12), biopsies were taken. In 0% (0/2) of TNO cases, biopsies were taken. The most common diagnosis of outpatient OGD biopsies was EoE in 46% (5/11); in one patient, the diagnosis was adenocarcinoma (Figure 4).

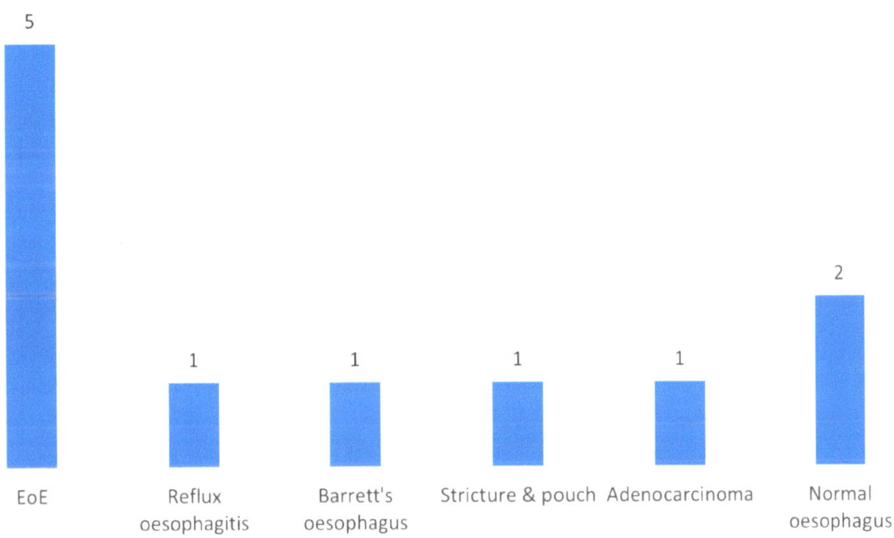

Figure 4. A number of patients with a diagnosis of outpatient OGD biopsies. EoE–eosinophilic oesophagitis.

When biopsies were performed during the inpatient and outpatient OGDs, in 71% (22/31), an insufficient number of oesophageal biopsies was taken (too few and/or from less than three levels of the oesophagus); therefore, only 29% of OGD biopsies were taken appropriately to diagnose or to exclude EoE.

In 53% of patients newly diagnosed with EoE, a specific number of eosinophils was not mentioned in their biopsy reports. Instead, pathologists used words such as 'mild/marked/predominant/dense infiltration of eosinophils' or similar.

In summary, when oesophageal biopsies were taken during the inpatient and outpatient OGDs, EoE was diagnosed in 48% (15/31) of patients. The mean age of these patients with newly diagnosed EoE was 28 years (range 15–60). The male to female ratio was 1.8:1. Animal-based food was the food bolus type in 100% of these EoE patients.

4. Discussion

This study has clearly shown that the majority of patients were under-investigated to rule out or diagnose EoE, the most common cause of FBO. When OGD was performed, only 29% had the recommended six biopsies taken. Despite this deficiency, our study still found 15 patients with EoE, but many more were likely missed due to failure to take adequate biopsies in all cases.

Males tend to be admitted with FBO more commonly compared to females [3,5]. This could be due to underlying pathology, such as EoE, which has been reported to be more common in males, and/or diet habits, such as higher quantities of meat being consumed by males [7,8]. In our cohort, males were admitted more commonly and were younger than females.

More admissions during the summer season and winter months may be explained due to dietary changes, including the increased consumption of barbeque meat during summer months and roasted meat during winter festive months. Similarly, increased admissions over weekends and Mondays may be associated with the higher consumption of meat when dining out. Previously, reports have suggested that increased FBO during summer months is due to increased levels of aeroallergens [9].

In our study, almost half of FBO cases resolved spontaneously, which is similar to a case series reported by Tsikoudas et al.—54% of 37 patients with symptoms of FBO for longer than 24 h found that the obstruction resolved spontaneously [10].

Different parenteral treatments may be given to relax different levels of oesophageal muscles such as benzodiazepines, glucagon, calcium channel blockers, and hyoscine butylbromide, the latter being the one we use in our hospital; nevertheless, we did not investigate the therapeutic effects of parenteral treatment for FBO. As there is no good evidence for any of these muscle relaxants in FBO, it might just be a UK-based ENT preference [11,12].

Instrumenting the oesophagus to resolve FBO can result in complications. In our cohort, one patient instrumented with RO and one with OGD had oesophageal tears, showing a two-fold higher complication rate with RO. Similarly, Straumann et al. reported a 20% (2/10) incidence of oesophageal tears with RO and 0% (0/124) with flexible endoscopy when removing a food bolus obstructing the oesophagus specifically in EoE patients [13]. Nevertheless, a meta-analysis by Ferrari et al. revealed no statistical significance of complication rates between flexible or rigid oesophagoscopy [14].

A general anaesthetic is required to perform all ROs, as well as during OGD/TNO if patients are not cooperative or if there is a high risk of aspiration [2]. Although our hospital follows guidelines on which speciality to refer the patients with FBO to, depending on whether it is above or below the sternal notch, the area of discomfort in the neck or chest often does not correlate with the site of obstruction [2,4]. In our ENT Department, the choice of intervention was decided based on the patients pointing out where the food was stuck. If they pointed in the neck and emergency theatres were available, then we performed RO. But if they pointed behind the sternum or emergency theatres were not available for RO within 8 h, then OGD was organised. Occasionally, a combined approach with OGD and RO might be required. In our cohort, one patient required a combined approach due to cervical osteophytes.

In our cohort, biopsies were taken in 48% (20/42) of inpatient OGDs, which is something that should be focused on in the future—taking biopsies in close to 100% of OGDs when performed for the removal of a soft food bolus. In a small group of our patients, OGDs with biopsies were arranged as a follow-up procedure if they were not performed during the inpatient stay, but 25% of our patients did not attend the arranged follow-up OGD; therefore, the aim should be to take biopsies during the index OGD. If a concern is prolonging the procedure due to taking biopsies, therefore making the procedure intolerable for patients, the operating endoscopists should highly consider performing the OGD under general anaesthetic.

Biopsies of the upper, middle, and lower oesophagus can be performed safely with OGD or TNO, both of which are flexible scopes. In our cohort, EoE was the most common diagnosis from biopsies taken during OGD, at 48% (15/31), with adenocarcinoma at 3% (1/31). A biopsy report of a 'normal oesophagus' cannot be considered unless six or more biopsies from three levels of the oesophagus have been taken [12].

As the commonest underlying oesophageal pathology presenting with FBO is EoE, these patients should be managed by GI doctors who can perform OGD to remove food boluses and take oesophageal biopsies to exclude EoE [5]. Since the results of this study were presented at multiple meetings, all FBO patients presenting at our hospital are admitted under GI doctors, as they are ultimately involved in looking after EoE patients. If in some hospitals, due to logistical reasons, FBO admissions are managed by ENT, then outpatient OGD or TNO with biopsies should be arranged for all patients as a follow-up investigation to look for the underlying cause of FBO. ENT should be involved in FBO cases presenting with an airway compromise or when the FBO is high in the oesophagus, preventing the OGD from advancing into the oesophagus.

In our cohort, 54% of patients (54/100) did not have a follow-up arranged. In 44% (20/46) of patients, appropriate follow-up with OGD or TNO was arranged, although the appointments did not take place in 30% (6/20) for unknown reasons (such as cancellation by patients or administrative error). Our findings highlight that the diagnosis of EoE was not considered in the majority of patients admitted to our unit with FBO. This has already been discussed in a systematic review by Bahgat et al. in 2015, but the practice has not improved since then, and further efforts to change the standards of investigation should be undertaken [15]. EoE is becoming a common disease and the number of patients with EoE as the cause of their FBO will rise as the disease itself becomes commoner [16].

5. Conclusions

Our retrospective study revealed that the focus of FBO admissions under the care of ENT was to resolve acute oesophageal obstruction. There was less focus on investigating the underlying oesophageal pathology. Patients with FBO should ideally be admitted under the care of GI doctors or upper GI surgeons, as they can perform OGD to resolve acute FBO and can examine the entire length of the oesophagus and take the appropriate number of biopsies. When patients are admitted under ENT care, ENT surgeons should be aware of EoE being the most common oesophageal pathology predisposing patients to FBO; therefore, patients should be referred for OGD or TNO with biopsies.

Author Contributions: Conceptualization, R.M.; methodology, R.M. and S.M.; formal analysis, R.M. and A.K.; resources, R.M.; data curation, R.M.; writing—original draft preparation, R.M.; writing—review and editing, R.M., A.K., M.M. and S.M.; visualisation, R.M.; supervision, M.M. and S.M. All authors have read and agreed to the published version of the manuscript.

Funding: This research received no external funding.

Institutional Review Board Statement: The study was conducted in accordance with the Declaration of Helsinki and approved by NHS Tayside Information Governance Caldicott Guardian (IGTCAL7909 on 6 July 2020).

Informed Consent Statement: Patient consent was waived due to this being a retrospective study, and it was approved by the NHS Tayside Information Governance Caldicott Guardian.

Data Availability Statement: Data are unavailable due to NHS Tayside privacy concerns, but, if required, the corresponding author will contact the NHS Tayside Information Governance Department with a request to share anonymized data.

Conflicts of Interest: R.M. has served on the advisory board on management pathways of food bolus obstruction and eosinophilic oesophagitis organised by Dr. Falk Pharma. M.M. is an advisory board member for Dr. Falk Pharma. A.K. and S.M. declare no relevant conflicts of interest.

Abbreviations

The following abbreviations are used in this manuscript:

ASGEE	American Society for Gastrointestinal Endoscopy
ENT	Ear, nose, and throat
EoE	Eosinophilic oesophagitis
ESGE	European Society of Gastrointestinal Endoscopy
FBO	Food bolus obstruction
GI	Gastroenterologists
GP	General Practitioners
Hpf	High power field
OGD	Oesophagogastroduodenoscopy
RO	Rigid oesophagoscopy
TNO	Transnasal oesophagoscopy
UK	United Kingdom

References

1. Hardman, J.; Sharma, N.; Smith, J.; Nankivell, P. Conservative management of oesophageal soft food bolus impaction. *Cochrane Database Syst. Rev.* **2020**, *5*, Cd007352. [CrossRef] [PubMed]
2. Birk, M.; Bauerfeind, P.; Deprez, P.H.; Häfner, M.; Hartmann, D.; Hassan, C.; Hucl, T.; Lesur, G.; Aabakken, L.; Meining, A. Removal of foreign bodies in the upper gastrointestinal tract in adults: European Society of Gastrointestinal Endoscopy (ESGE) Clinical Guideline. *Endoscopy* **2016**, *48*, 489–496. [CrossRef] [PubMed]
3. Ntuli, Y.; Bough, I.; Wilson, M. Recognising eosinophilic oesophagitis as a cause of food bolus obstruction. *Frontline Gastroenterol.* **2020**, *11*, 11–15. [CrossRef] [PubMed]
4. Stubington, T.J.; Kamani, T. Food bolus and oesophageal foreign body: A summary of the evidence and proposed management process. *Eur. Arch. Otorhinolaryngol.* **2021**, *278*, 3613–3623. [CrossRef] [PubMed]
5. Attwood, S.E. Overview of eosinophilic oesophagitis. *Br. J. Hosp. Med.* **2019**, *80*, 132–138. [CrossRef] [PubMed]
6. Lucendo, A.J.; Molina-Infante, J.; Arias, Á.; von Arnim, U.; Bredenoord, A.J.; Bussmann, C.; Dias, J.A.; Bove, M.; González-Cervera, J.; Larsson, H.; et al. Guidelines on eosinophilic esophagitis: Evidence-based statements and recommendations for diagnosis and management in children and adults. *United Eur. Gastroenterol. J.* **2017**, *5*, 335–358. [CrossRef] [PubMed]
7. Feraco, A.; Armani, A.; Amoah, I.; Guseva, E.; Camajani, E.; Gorini, S.; Strollo, R.; Padua, E.; Caprio, M.; Lombardo, M. Assessing gender differences in food preferences and physical activity: A population-based survey. *Front. Nutr.* **2024**, *11*, 1348456. [CrossRef] [PubMed]
8. Lombardo, M.; Feraco, A.; Camajani, E.; Gorini, S.; Strollo, R.; Armani, A.; Padua, E.; Caprio, M. Effects of Different Nutritional Patterns and Physical Activity on Body Composition: A Gender and Age Group Comparative Study. *Foods* **2024**, *13*, 529. [CrossRef] [PubMed]
9. Philpott, H.L.; Nandurkar, S.; Thien, F.; Bloom, S.; Lin, E.; Goldberg, R.; Boyapati, R.; Finch, A.; Royce, S.G.; Gibson, P.R. Seasonal recurrence of food bolus obstruction in eosinophilic esophagitis. *Intern. Med. J.* **2015**, *45*, 939–943. [CrossRef] [PubMed]
10. Tsikoudas, A.; Kochillas, X.; Kelleher, R.J.; Mills, R. The management of acute oesophageal obstruction from a food bolus. Can we be more conservative? *Eur. Arch. Otorhinolaryngol.* **2005**, *262*, 528–530. [CrossRef] [PubMed]
11. Price, T.; Jones, S.E.; Montgomery, P.Q. Is current UK management of oesophageal food bolus obstruction evidence based? An e-mail survey and literature review. *Eur. Arch. Otorhinolaryngol.* **2007**, *264*, 329–335. [CrossRef] [PubMed]
12. Dhar, A.; Haboubi, H.N.; Attwood, S.E.; Auth, M.K.H.; Dunn, J.M.; Sweis, R.; Morris, D.; Epstein, J.; Novelli, M.R.; Hunter, H.; et al. British Society of Gastroenterology (BSG) and British Society of Paediatric Gastroenterology, Hepatology and Nutrition (BSPGHAN) joint consensus guidelines on the diagnosis and management of eosinophilic oesophagitis in children and adults. *Gut* **2022**, *71*, 1459–1487. [CrossRef] [PubMed]
13. Straumann, A.; Bussmann, C.; Zuber, M.; Vannini, S.; Simon, H.-U.; Schoepfer, A. Eosinophilic esophagitis: Analysis of food impaction and perforation in 251 adolescent and adult patients. *Clin. Gastroenterol. Hepatol.* **2008**, *6*, 598–600. [CrossRef] [PubMed]

14. Ferrari, D.; Aiolfi, A.; Bonitta, G.; Riva, C.G.; Rausa, E.; Siboni, S.; Toti, F.; Bonavina, L. Flexible versus rigid endoscopy in the management of esophageal foreign body impaction: Systematic review and meta-analysis. *World J. Emerg. Surg.* **2018**, *13*, 42. [CrossRef] [PubMed]
15. Bahgat, M.; Dawe, N.; Flood, L. Eosinophilic oesophagitis: A systematic review for otolaryngologists. *J. Laryngol. Otol.* **2015**, *129*, 1156–1166. [CrossRef] [PubMed]
16. Limketkai, B.N.; Shah, S.C.; Hirano, I.; Bellaguarda, E.; Colombel, J.-F. Epidemiology and implications of concurrent diagnosis of eosinophilic oesophagitis and IBD based on a prospective population-based analysis. *Gut* **2019**, *68*, 2152–2160. [CrossRef] [PubMed]

medicina

MDPI

Article

An Important Biomarker in Patients with Bell's Palsy: Serum Calprotectin

Cihan Türker [1], Elif Emre [2], Süleyman Aydın [3], Mustafa Dalgıç [4,*] and Deniz Baklacı [5]

1 Department of Otolaryngology, Private Medical Hospital, Elazig 23040, Turkey; cihan_turker23@hotmail.com
2 Department of Anatomy, Firat University Faculty of Medicine, Elazig 23200, Turkey; elifkaplan1.1@gmail.com
3 Department of Biochemistry, Firat University Faculty of Medicine, Elazig 23200, Turkey; saydin1@firat.edu.tr
4 Department of Otolaryngology, Ataturk State Hospital, Zonguldak 67030, Turkey
5 Department of Otolaryngology, Bulent Ecevit University Faculty of Medicine, Zonguldak 67000, Turkey; doktorent@gmail.com
* Correspondence: dalgic_816@hotmail.com; Tel.: +90-5427149385; Fax: +90-3722612388

Abstract: *Background and Objectives*: This study aimed to examine the relationship between serum calprotectin levels and facial paralysis in patients with Bell's palsy and to determine its prognostic significance. *Materials and Methods*: This study included 40 patients diagnosed with Bell's palsy and 20 healthy individuals as controls. The patients were categorized into three groups based on their response to treatment: complete response, partial response, and no response. Blood samples were taken before treatment and in the third month after treatment to measure C-reactive protein, white blood cell count, lymphocyte count, neutrophil count, neutrophil-to-lymphocyte ratio, and calprotectin levels. *Results*: Serum calprotectin levels were found to be elevated in patients with BP compared to the healthy controls; however, no significant correlation was observed between calprotectin levels and disease prognosis. *Conclusions*: The findings suggest that Bell's palsy patients have elevated serum calprotectin levels compared to healthy individuals, indicating the potential use of calprotectin as a biomarker in Bell's palsy. However, no significant difference in calprotectin levels was observed between patients with varying degrees of treatment response, suggesting that calprotectin may be limited in predicting disease prognosis.

Keywords: Bell's palsy; calprotectin; marker

1. Introduction

Acute peripheral facial paralysis (APFP) is characterized by acute-onset facial nerve paralysis, typically affecting one side of the face. Idiopathic peripheral facial paralysis, commonly known as Bell's palsy (BP), accounts for approximately 70% of APFP cases and occurs with similar frequency among men and women [1]. Although the exact mechanism of BP remains unclear, it is thought to be related to the reactivation of herpes simplex virus type 1 or varicella-zoster virus. In addition to viral factors, tumors, trauma, anatomical anomalies, inflammation, ischemia, and cold exposure have also been implicated as etiological factors [2].

The primary treatment of BP involves corticosteroids and antiviral medications, although the response to therapy varies. While the majority of patients experience full recovery within three to six months, there are cases where no recovery occurs [3]. Therefore, determining the prognosis of the disease is of critical importance.

The severity of facial paralysis is a key factor in predicting prognosis. The House–Brackmann and Sunnybrook grading systems are commonly used to assess the degree of paralysis. Electrophysiological modalities such as electroneurography, electromyography, and nerve stimulation tests are also employed to evaluate prognosis. Electroneurography is highly correlated with disease prognosis, providing an indication of facial nerve degeneration. It is particularly important for patients scheduled for facial nerve decompression. Electromyography and nerve stimulation tests are auxiliary tools in predicting prognosis; however, these tests are typically conducted at least three days after symptom onset [4]. Thus, there is a need for additional biomarkers to predict facial paralysis prognosis earlier. To this end, various inflammatory, metabolic, and hematological markers have been investigated [5,6].

Inflammatory causes have been implicated in the etiology of BP. According to the inflammation theory, the facial nerve becomes inflamed, causing swelling of the nerve sheath, which can lead to entrapment in the labyrinthine segment, resulting in paralysis [7]. Several studies have thus examined various inflammatory markers and immune system cells in patients with BP. Among the most frequently examined parameters are the neutrophil-to-lymphocyte ratio (NLR), C-reactive protein (CRP), albumin, and procalcitonin.

Calprotectin is a major antimicrobial protein belonging to the S100 family of proteins. It enters the systemic circulation during inflammation through neutrophil activation or the adhesion of monocytes to the epithelium, and is therefore considered an inflammatory biomarker [8].

This study aimed to explore the relationship between serum calprotectin levels and facial paralysis in patients diagnosed with BP and to determine its prognostic significance.

2. Materials and Methods

2.1. Study Design

A retrospective study was carried out, between 1 January 2023 and 30 June 2024, within a tertiary referral center hospital. This study included 40 patients diagnosed with BP, as well as a control group of 20 healthy individuals. A complete ear–nose–throat and head and neck examinations were performed for all patients. Complete blood count (CBC), serum calprotectin, pure tone audiometry, stapes reflex, routine blood biochemistry, and viral serological markers were obtained from the patients diagnosed with unilateral peripheral facial paralysis in order to exclude any other causes of facial paralysis. Additionally, contrast-enhanced MRI and temporal CT were obtained from all patients at the onset of the treatment. The diagnosis of Bell's palsy was confirmed by at least two otolaryngology specialists in the patient group. In the control group, the CBC was obtained and no other tests were performed.

2.2. Inclusion and Exclusion Criteria

This study included 40 patients diagnosed with BP who were treated at a tertiary referral center hospital, as well as a control group of 20 healthy individuals. All patients underwent full head and neck examination, and other causes of facial palsy were excluded. This study included patients with unilateral peripheral facial palsy that developed rapidly (within 72 h) and had no other identifiable causes. Patients with any autoimmune disease, rheumatologic disease, acute or chronic infection, cardiovascular disease, diabetes mellitus, metabolic syndrome, chronic obstructive pulmonary disease, amyloidosis, chronic renal failure, obstructive sleep apnea, active smoking, or Otological diseases were excluded from this study. The control group consisted of healthy volunteers without ear pathology or systemic disorder and with normal audiological findings.

2.3. Study Setting and Population

The patient group consisted of 20 males and 20 females, while the control group included 10 males and 10 females. The mean age was 44.17 ± 18.33 years in the BP group and 44.50 ± 10.72 years in the control group. The patients were administered a standard treatment protocol consisting of steroids and antiviral drugs. The patients in the BP group were further divided into three subgroups based on their response to treatment: complete response, partial response, and no response. Blood samples were taken from the patients before treatment and at the third month of follow-up to measure CRP, white blood cell (WBC) count, lymphocyte count, neutrophil count, NLR, and calprotectin levels. These values were compared within the BP group and with the values obtained from the healthy control group. The effect of inflammatory markers on patient prognosis was also investigated.

2.4. Blood Sampling

All blood samples were drawn by same personnel and immediately analyzed without any delay. The Beckman Coulter LH 750 automated complete blood analyzer device (Beckman Coulter, Pasadena, CA, USA) was used to analyze complete blood count (CBC) parameters. Calprotectin was analyzed with a ChroMate, Microplate Reader P4300 devices (Awareness Technology Instruments, Palm City, FL, USA), and the results were reported in ng/mL.

2.5. Methods of Data Collection

Data were collected between 1 January 2023 and 30 June 2024. All data were collected and organized in a structured database using Microsoft Excel. Data entry was performed by trained personnel. Our database was regularly checked for any missing or inconsistent data. Data analyses were conducted based on the data stored in this Excel database.

2.6. Statistical Analysis

Descriptive statistics for continuous data were presented as mean ± standard deviation, median, minimum, and maximum values, while categorical data were presented as numbers and percentages. The Shapiro–Wilk test was used to assess the normality of the distribution of continuous variables. The Mann–Whitney U test was employed to compare continuous data between two groups. The Wilcoxon test was used to compare pre- and post-treatment measurements within the patient group. The Chi-square test was applied for group comparisons of nominal variables (in cross-tables). IBM SPSS version 20 (Chicago, IL, USA) was used for statistical analyses, with statistical significance set at $p < 0.05$.

3. Results

The mean age of the BP group was 44.17 ± 18.33 years, similar to the control group's mean of 44.50 ± 10.72 years ($p = 0.815$). No significant difference was observed in gender distribution between the two groups ($p > 0.05$) (Table 1). Except for Bell's palsy, the patients were otherwise healthy.

CRP levels significantly decreased after treatment compared to pre-treatment values ($p < 0.001$), as did WBC counts ($p < 0.001$). However, there was no significant change in lymphocyte levels ($p > 0.05$). Neutrophil counts and NLR were also significantly lower after treatment ($p < 0.01$ and $p < 0.05$, respectively) (Table 2). Similarly, calprotectin levels showed a significant reduction after treatment ($p < 0.001$) (Figure 1).

Table 1. Comparison of age and gender between the BP and control groups.

	BP Group (*n* = 40)	Control Group (*n* = 20)	*p* Value
Age (year), mean ± SD (Min–Max)	44.17 ± 18.33 (14–74)	44.50 ± 10.72 (15–64)	0.815 [a]
Gender, n (%)			
Male	20 (50)	10 (50)	4.72 [b]
Female	20 (50)	10 (50)	

[a] Mann–Whitney U test, [b] Chi-square test, BP: Bell's palsy, SD: standard deviation.

Table 2. Comparison of pre- and post-treatment measurements in the BP group.

	Pre-Treatment	Post-Treatment	
	Mean ± SD Median (Min–Max)	Mean ± SD Median (Min–Max)	*p* *
CRP	3.00 ± 2.77 2.5 (0.2–11)	1.36 ± 1.36 1.05 (0–6.4)	<0.001
WBC count	10.94 ± 4.15 10.42 (6.49–20.94)	7.75 ± 1.62 7.40 (5.24–11.33)	<0.001
Lymphocyte count	2.17 ± 1.05 2.19 (0.67–4.37)	1.91 ± 0.58 1.90 (1.03–2.87)	0.519
Neutrophil count	8.16 ± 4.31 7.48 (3.30–18.94)	5.34 ± 1.77 5.08 (2.16–9.04)	0.001
Neutrophil-to-lymphocyte ratio	5.29 ± 4.18 4.17 (1.10–13.31)	3.20 ± 1.89 2.91 (0.86–8.29)	0.038
Calprotectin	29.94 ± 21.49 24.19 (5.61–73.46)	14.45 ± 9.91 9.90 (2.80–35.32)	<0.001
Stage	3 (2–4)	2 (1–3)	<0.001

* Wilcoxon test, BP: Bell's palsy, SD: standard deviation, CRP: C-reactive protein, WBC: white blood cell.

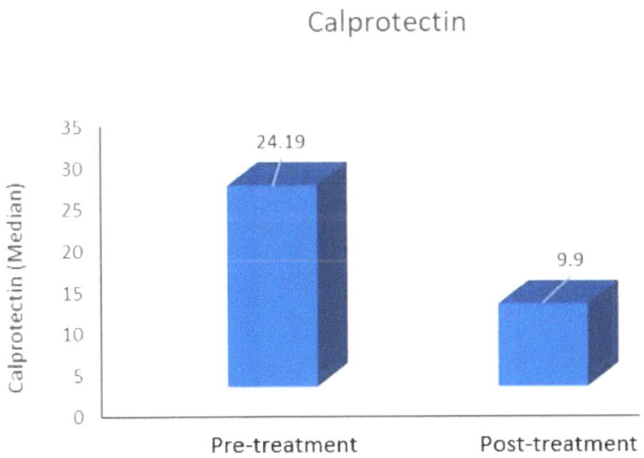

Figure 1. Pre- and post-treatment calprotectin values of patients with Bell's palsy.

When comparing pre-treatment values between the BP and control groups, WBC counts ($p < 0.001$), neutrophil counts ($p < 0.001$), NLR ($p < 0.01$), and calprotectin levels ($p < 0.05$) were significantly higher in the BP group, while CRP and lymphocyte values did not differ significantly ($p > 0.05$) (Table 3).

Table 3. Comparison of pre-treatment laboratory parameters between the BP and control groups.

Pre-Treatment Parameter	BP Group (n = 40) Mean ± SD Median (Min–Max)	Control (n = 20) Mean ± SD Median (Min–Max)	p *
CRP	3.00 ± 2.77 2.5 (0.2–11)	2.05 ± 1.89 1.95 (0.2–9.5)	0.322
WBC count	10.94 ± 4.15 10.42 (6.49–20.94)	7.01 ± 1.43 7 (4.80–9.34)	<0.001
Lymphocyte count	2.17 ± 1.05 2.19 (0.67–4.37)	2.17 ± 0.68 2.01 (1.49–3.64)	0.975
Neutrophil count	8.16 ± 4.31 7.48 (3.30–18.94)	3.92 ± 1.42 3.52 (2.37–6.72)	<0.001
Neutrophil-to-lymphocyte ratio	5.29 ± 4.18 4.17 (1.10–13.31)	2.03 ± 0.93 1.93 (0.81–3.65)	0.007
Calprotectin	29.94 ± 21.49 24.19 (5.61–73.46)	14.35 ± 7.72 14.69 (2.19–29.40)	0.012

* Mann–Whitney U test, BP: Bell's palsy, SD: standard deviation, CRP: C-reactive protein, WBC: white blood cell.

Post-treatment comparisons revealed that the BP group had lower CRP levels than the control group ($p < 0.05$) and higher neutrophil counts ($p < 0.01$) and NLR ($p < 0.05$). No significant differences were observed in post-treatment WBC or lymphocyte counts or calprotectin levels between the two groups ($p > 0.05$).

Following treatment, 18 patients (45%) in the BP group achieved full recovery, 15 (37.5%) showed partial recovery, and 7 (17.5%) did not respond to treatment. The calprotectin levels of the BP group did not significantly differ between patients with complete response, partial response, or no response, either before or after treatment ($p > 0.05$ for both) (Table 4).

Table 4. Comparison of pre- and post-treatment calprotectin levels according to treatment response in the BP group.

	Complete Response (n = 18) Mean ± SD Median (Min–Max)	Partial/No Response (n = 22) Mean ± SD Median (Min–Max)	p *
Pre-treatment calprotectin	33.46 ± 23.95 27.94 (7.48–73.46)	27.06 ± 19.34 22.06 (5.61–66.02)	0.381
Post-treatment calprotectin	12.21 ± 10.91 8.77 (2.8–35.32)	16.29 ± 8.85 15.23 (4.44–30.02)	0.089

* Mann–Whitney U test, BP: Bell's palsy, SD: standard deviation.

4. Discussion

Inflammatory causes are considered significant in the pathogenesis of BP [7]. Accordingly, several studies have examined the relationship between BP and immune system cells and biomarkers, focusing primarily on lymphocytes, neutrophils, monocytes, and cellular immune responses [9]. Research indicates elevated levels of inflammatory markers, such as interleukin-1 (IL-1), IL-6, IL-8, and tumor necrosis factor-α, in patients with BP [10,11]. Furthermore, NLR has been shown to increase significantly in patients with BP, and its relevance in predicting disease prognosis has been emphasized. Studies have also reported that NLR is higher in patients with BP who have not fully recovered compared to those who have achieved complete recovery, suggesting that NLR can be used to predict prognosis in BP [12,13]. Supporting these findings, the current study revealed a significant decrease in NLR after treatment compared to pre-treatment values ($p < 0.05$). Additionally, post-treatment NLR values in the BP group were significantly higher than those in the control group ($p < 0.05$).

In a study by Kim et al., patients who did not respond fully to treatment had lower WBC and eosinophil counts after seven days of therapy than those with a complete treatment response. Similarly, lower lymphocyte counts were observed in non-responders before and after seven days of treatment compared to complete responders [14]. In contrast, our study found no statistically significant difference in lymphocyte levels before and after treatment ($p > 0.05$). Furthermore, no significant difference was observed between post-treatment lymphocyte levels between the BP and control groups ($p > 0.05$).

In recent years, studies exploring the relationship between serum calprotectin levels and otolaryngological diseases have increased in number. One study found a correlation between symptom severity and serum calprotectin levels in patients with chronic rhinosinusitis [15]. In another study, Kuzucu et al. demonstrated higher serum calprotectin levels in patients diagnosed with idiopathic sudden sensorineural hearing loss compared to healthy individuals. The authors also reported higher calprotectin levels in patients who did not respond to treatment compared to those with partial or full recovery, suggesting that serum calprotectin may be a marker of disease severity and treatment response in idiopathic sudden sensorineural hearing loss [16].

In a study by Van Crombruggen et al., patients with chronic rhinosinusitis and nasal polyposis exhibited higher serum calprotectin levels than the healthy population. The authors suggested that this finding could be attributed to the release of calprotectin from cells due to inflammation [17]. Similarly, Erdoğan et al. reported higher serum calprotectin levels in patients with nasal polyposis compared to healthy controls. They suggested that elevated serum calprotectin served as a robust marker of nasal inflammation and could predict a greater need for nasal and systemic steroid therapy, independent of physical examination or computed tomography findings [18]. Kum et al. demonstrated that patients with obstructive sleep apnea had higher serum calprotectin levels than healthy individuals, and these levels also correlated with the severity of obstructive sleep apnea [19].

In this study, pre-treatment levels of CRP, WBC, neutrophils, NLR, and serum calprotectin were significantly higher in patients with BP compared to their post-treatment values ($p < 0.05$). No significant difference was found in lymphocyte levels before and after treatment ($p > 0.05$). Additionally, pre-treatment levels of CRP, WBC, neutrophils, NLR, and serum calprotectin were higher in patients with BP compared to the healthy population ($p < 0.05$), while lymphocyte levels showed no significant difference ($p > 0.05$). Furthermore, no significant difference was observed in calprotectin levels between patients who achieved full recovery, partial recovery, or no response, either before or after treatment ($p > 0.05$).

Our study is the first in the literature to investigate the relationship between BP and serum calprotectin levels. The findings suggest that BP patients have elevated serum calprotectin levels compared to healthy individuals, indicating the potential use of calprotectin as a biomarker in BP. However, no significant difference in calprotectin levels was observed between patients with varying degrees of treatment response, suggesting that calprotectin may be limited in predicting disease prognosis.

5. Conclusions

This study showed elevated serum calprotectin levels in patients with BP compared to the healthy population. However, no significant correlation was found between calprotectin levels and disease prognosis.

Author Contributions: Conceptualization, M.D. and D.B.; methodology, C.T.; software, E.E.; validation, S.A., C.T., and E.E.; formal analysis, M.D.; investigation, D.B., M.D., C.T., E.E., and S.A.; resources, S.A.; data curation, E.E. and C.T.; writing—original draft preparation, M.D. and D.B.; writing—review and editing, M.D. and D.B.; visualization, S.A.; supervision, D.B. and S.A. All authors have read and agreed to the published version of the manuscript.

Funding: This research received no external funding.

Institutional Review Board Statement: This study was conducted in accordance with the Declaration of Helsinki and approved by the Firat University Non-Interventional Research Ethics Committee (protocol no. 2021/01-20 approval date: 14 January 2021).

Informed Consent Statement: Informed consent was obtained from all subjects involved in this study.

Data Availability Statement: The original contributions presented in this study are included in the article. Further inquiries can be directed to the corresponding author.

Conflicts of Interest: The authors declare no conflicts of interest.

References

1. Singh, A.; Deshmukh, P. Bell's Palsy: A Review. *Cureus* **2022**, *14*, e30186. [CrossRef] [PubMed]
2. Zhang, W.; Xu, L.; Luo, T.; Wu, F.; Zhao, B.; Li, X. The etiology of Bell's palsy: A review. *J. Neurol.* **2020**, *267*, 1896–1905. [CrossRef] [PubMed]
3. Wasano, K.; Ishikawa, T.; Kawasaki, T.; Yamamoto, S.; Tomisato, S.; Shinden, S.; Minami, S.; Wakabayashi, T.; Ogawa, K. Novel pre-therapeutic scoring system using patient and haematological data to predict facial palsy prognosis. *Clin. Otolaryngol.* **2017**, *42*, 1224–1228. [CrossRef] [PubMed]
4. Lee, D.H. Clinical Efficacy of Electroneurography in Acute Facial Paralysis. *J. Audiol. Otol.* **2016**, *20*, 8–12. [CrossRef] [PubMed]
5. Babademez, M.A.; Gul, F.; Kale, H.; Muderris, T.; Bayazit, Y.; Ergin, M.; Erel, O.; Kiris, M. Thiol/disulphide homeostasis in Bell's palsy as a novel pathogenetic marker. *Clin. Otolaryngol.* **2017**, *42*, 239–244. [CrossRef] [PubMed]
6. Oya, R.; Takenaka, Y.; Imai, T.; Sato, T.; Oshima, K.; Ohta, Y.; Inohara, H. Neutrophil-to-Lymphocyte Ratio and Platelet-to-Lymphocyte Ratio as Prognostic Hematologic Markers of Bell's Palsy: A Meta-analysis. *Otol. Neurotol.* **2019**, *40*, 681–687. [CrossRef] [PubMed]
7. Kefalidis, G.; Riga, M.; Argyropoulou, P.; Katotomichelakis, M.; Gouveris, C.; Prassopoulos, P.; Danielides, V. Is the width of the labyrinthine portion of the fallopian tube implicated in the pathophysiology of Bell's palsy?: A prospective clinical study using computed tomography. *Laryngoscope* **2010**, *120*, 1203–1207. [CrossRef] [PubMed]
8. Kim, T.H.; Yeo, S.G.; Byun, J.Y. Role of Biomarkers as Prognostic Factors in Acute Peripheral Facial Palsy. *Int. J. Mol. Sci.* **2021**, *23*, 307. [CrossRef] [PubMed]
9. Kiliçkaya, M.M.; Tuz, M.; Yariktaş, M.; Yasan, H.; Aynalı, G.; Bagci, Ö. The Importance of the Neutrophil-Lymphocyte Ratio in Patients with Idiopathic Peripheral Facial Palsy. *Int. J. Otolaryngol.* **2015**, *2015*, 981950. [CrossRef] [PubMed]
10. Greco, A.; Gallo, A.; Fusconi, M.; Marinelli, C.; Macri, G.F.; de Vincentiis, M. Bell's palsy and autoimmunity. *Autoimmun. Rev.* **2012**, *12*, 323–328. [CrossRef] [PubMed]
11. Yilmaz, M.; Tarakcioglu, M.; Bayazit, N.; Bayazit, Y.A.; Namiduru, M.; Kanlikama, M. Serum cytokine levels in Bell's palsy. *J. Neurol. Sci.* **2002**, *197*, 69–72. [CrossRef] [PubMed]
12. Kum, R.O.; Yurtsever Kum, N.; Ozcan, M.; Yilmaz, Y.F.; Gungor, V.; Unal, A.; Ciliz, D.S. Elevated neutrophil-to-lymphocyte ratio in Bell's palsy and its correlation with facial nerve enhancement on MRI. *Otolaryngol. Head Neck Surg.* **2015**, *152*, 130–135. [CrossRef] [PubMed]
13. Bucak, A.; Ulu, S.; Oruc, S.; Yucedag, F.; Tekin, M.S.; Karakaya, F.; Aycicek, A. Neutrophil-to-lymphocyte ratio as a novel-potential marker for predicting prognosis of Bell palsy. *Laryngoscope* **2014**, *124*, 1678–1681. [CrossRef] [PubMed]
14. Kim, S.J.; Lee, H.Y. Hematological Findings in Patients with Acute Peripheral Facial Palsy. *J. Int. Adv. Otol.* **2020**, *16*, 382–386. [CrossRef] [PubMed]
15. Candar, T.; Baklaci, D.; Kuzucu, I.; Kayabasi, S. A proinflammatory marker in chronic rhinosinusitis: Serum calprotectin. *Acta Biochim. Pol.* **2020**, *67*, 367–371. [CrossRef] [PubMed]
16. Kuzucu, İ.; Çandar, T.; Baklacı, D.; Güler, İ.; Kum, R.O.; Arslan, H.; Özcan, M. A Prognostic Marker in Idiopathic Sudden Sensorineural Hearing Loss: Serum Calprotectin. *Clin. Exp. Otorhinolaryngol.* **2020**, *13*, 36–40. [CrossRef] [PubMed]
17. Van Crombruggen, K.; Vogl, T.; Pérez-Novo, C.; Holtappels, G.; Bachert, C. Differential release and deposition of S100A8/A9 proteins in inflamed upper airway tissue. *Eur. Respir. J.* **2016**, *47*, 264–274. [CrossRef] [PubMed]

18. Erdoğan, A.M.; Özdaş, T.; Çakır, A.; Alagoz, S.; Bal, K.K.; Gorgulu, O.; Kuran, G.; Matyar, S.; Gorgulu, F.F. Predictive value of serum calprotectin level in nasal polyposis. *B-ENT* **2023**, *19*, 151–156. [CrossRef]
19. Kum, N.Y.; Kum, R.O.; Candar, T.; Baklaci, D.; Guler, I.; Kuzucu, I.; Ozcan Kursat Murat Ozcan, M.; Dere, H. Elevated serum calprotectin as an inflammatory marker in obstructive sleep apnea. *Cranio J. Craniomandib. Sleep Pract.* **2020**, *41*, 160–166. [CrossRef]

medicina

MDPI

Article

Flexible Nasendoscopy in Stevens–Johnson Syndrome/Toxic Epidermal Necrolysis: A Ten-Year Otolaryngology Experience

Matthew Min Xian Yii [1,*], Antonia Rowson [1], Milan van Ammers [2] and Jessica Prasad [1]

[1] Ear, Nose and Throat Department, Alfred Health, Melbourne, VIC 3004, Australia
[2] Eastern Health, Box Hill, VIC 3128, Australia
* Correspondence: matthew.mxy@gmail.com; Tel.: +61-437898102

Abstract: *Background and Objectives*: The primary objective of this study was to identify factors predictive of laryngeal involvement in patients with Stevens–Johnson syndrome/toxic epidermal necrolysis (SJS/TEN). The secondary objective was to observe the effect of laryngeal involvement upon short-term patient prognosis, including intensive care unit (ICU) stay and intubation rates. We present the largest cohort of patients examined for upper aerodigestive manifestations of SJS/TEN. *Materials and Methods*: We performed a retrospective observational analytic study of patients at a state-wide Australian Burns referral center between January 2013 to December 2022. Inclusion criteria were adult patients who underwent flexible nasendoscopy (FNE) with biopsy-proven SJS/TEN. Data collected from medical records included patient factors, aerodigestive symptoms, bedside examination, FNE findings, TEN-specific severity-of-illness score (SCORTEN) on admission, and patient outcomes such as intubation and ICU admission. *Results*: Fifty-four patients with biopsy-proven SJS/TEN underwent FNE, with 17 (31.5%) identified to have laryngeal involvement. Laryngeal involvement was not significantly associated with intubation, ICU stay, or mortality ($p > 0.05$). The presence of either aerodigestive symptoms or oral cavity involvement was highly sensitive (94.1%, 95% CI 73.0–99.7%) for laryngeal involvement. *Conclusions*: We did not find laryngeal involvement in SJS/TEN to significantly impact short-term outcomes, including intubation or mortality. FNE is the gold standard of upper aerodigestive assessment. Simple clinical evaluation of the oral cavity and a history of aerodigestive symptoms also provided a sensitive predictor of the laryngeal complications of SJS/TEN.

Keywords: Stevens–Johnson syndrome; toxic epidermal necrolysis; flexible nasendoscopy; airway

1. Introduction

Stevens–Johnson syndrome (SJS) and toxic epidermal necrolysis (TEN) exist on a spectrum of rare severe cutaneous immune-mediated adverse reactions in which extensive epidermal necrosis and mucositis occur [1]. SJS and TEN represent the same disease process but are differentiated by the extent of body surface area (BSA) involvement; SJS involves less than 10% BSA, SJS/TEN overlap 10–30% BSA, and TEN involves more than 30% BSA. The terms "SJS/TEN" and "epidermal necrolysis" encompass the spectrum of disease. This severe adverse reaction is usually triggered by medication [2], with release of cytotoxic proteins by drug-specific CD8+ T cells causing epidermal necrolysis [1].

An estimated incidence of five to six cases per million per year suffer SJS/TEN [3]. Female gender, increasing age, human immunodeficiency virus infection, connective tissue disease, malignancy, and certain human leukocyte antigen phenotype frequencies are risk factors for this disease [3,4]. Where medications are not causative, other precipitants include mycoplasma pneumonia and vaccination. A further 15–20% of cases remain idiopathic.

Widespread epidermal and mucosal involvement merits a routine multidisciplinary approach. Mucosal surfaces of the oral cavity (90%), nasal cavity (50%), ear (50%), and larynx (30%) are commonly affected [5]. Aerodigestive mucosal involvement may compromise the airway via oedema, hypersecretion, and inflammation, necessitating definitive airway management [6]. Otolaryngology input may be sought to assess upper aerodigestive involvement not assessable simply by anterior rhinoscopy or oral cavity examination. Flexible nasendoscopy (FNE) can be performed at the bedside with topical anesthetic to assess the larynx and hypopharynx [7]. FNE is the gold standard for diagnosis of laryngeal involvement of SJS/TEN; however, predictive factors for laryngeal involvement and the utility of assessment in predicting intubation are unknown [6]. Limited primary literature exists regarding the acute management of aerodigestive SJS/TEN and its impact upon a patient's admission.

The primary objective of this study is to determine factors predictive of laryngeal involvement. The secondary objective is to determine the influence of laryngeal involvement on patient prognosis, intensive care unit (ICU) stay, and rates of intubation.

2. Materials and Methods

We performed a retrospective observational analytic study of patients at a state-wide Australian burns referral center, drawing patients from a ten-year period between January 2013 and December 2022. Inclusion criteria were for patients at least 18 years of age at time of admission, who had a confirmed histologic diagnosis of SJS/TEN, and had undergone a FNE examination during their admission. Ethical approval was granted by the Alfred Health Research and Ethics Committee (approval number: 674/22).

Patients were identified via ear, nose, and throat (ENT) and burns unit audit data. Data were collated into a de-identified spreadsheet accessible only by researchers approved by the Alfred Health Research and Ethics Committee. Information gathered from medical records included age at time of admission, time from presentation to FNE, causative agent of SJS/TEN, total body surface area involved, area of desquamation, and TEN-specific severity-of-illness score (SCORTEN) on admission. Data points of aerodigestive assessment findings collected were dysphonia, stridor, dysphagia/odynophagia, and the presence of lip, oral cavity, or nasal cavity involvement. FNE findings collected were involvement of the nasopharynx, oropharynx, and/or larynx, and descriptors of subsites of these regions if involved. In patients who underwent repeat FNE, we documented whether findings worsened compared to initial assessment. Outcome data points collected were whether patients required intubation, cause for intubation, whether patients were admitted to ICU, length of ICU stay, length of hospital stay, and mortality.

SCORTEN is a validated severity-of-illness score applicable to patients with SJS/TEN [8]. It is calculated using seven prognostic factors, each scoring one point:

1. Age $\geq$ 40 years;
2. Heart rate $\geq$ 120 beats per minute;
3. Associated malignancy;
4. Detached body surface area $\geq$ 10%;
5. Serum urea > 10 mmol/L;
6. Serum bicarbonate < 20 mmol/L;
7. Serum glucose > 14 mmol/L.

Mortality rates increase with SCORTEN; a score $\geq$ 5 indicates a mortality rate of >90%. The majority of cases had SCORTEN documented on admission. For scores not explicitly documented, this was calculated at time of data collection from admission electronic medical record data and historical pathology results.

Statistical analysis was performed using GraphPad Prism 9. All continuous variables were found to be non-normally distributed on D'Agostino–Pearson testing. When comparing categorical variables with categorical outcomes (laryngeal involvement vs. intubation/ICU admission/mortality), Fisher's exact test was used due to the small sample size. The non-parametric Mann–Whitney U testing was used to determine categorical variables with continuous outcomes (laryngeal involvement vs. ICU/hospital length of stay). Sensitivity and specificity values with a 95% confidence interval (CI) were calculated using the Wilson/Brown method. Simple logistic regression was used to compare SCORTEN with the presence of laryngeal involvement. Statistical significance was set at $p < 0.05$.

3. Results

Sixty-seven adult patients were identified with biopsy-proven SJS/TEN over the relevant ten-year period. Fifty-four adult patients underwent FNE. Of the thirteen excluded patients, six were not referred to ENT, five were not scoped as they were intubated prior to review, one patient died prior to review, and one patient was assessed by ENT, but no FNE was performed.

The median age of patients meeting inclusion criteria was 57.5 (IQR 33.5–68.3) years (Table 1). Twenty-five patients (46.3%) were male, and 29 (53.7%) were female. The most common precipitants were antibiotics in twenty cases (37.0%), unknown cause in eleven (20.4%), and antiepileptics in seven (13.0%). The median time from either emergency department presentation or initial documented suspicion of SJS/TEN (if admitted prior to developing SJS/TEN) to FNE was 10.5 (IQR 2.8–24.0) hours. On admission/initial review for SJS/TEN, the median total body surface area of SJS/TEN was 40.0% (IQR 30.0–70.0%) and median body surface area of detachment was 11.0% (IQR 5.0–25.8%). SCORTEN 2 was the most common, accounting for 17 patients (31.5%) at initial review. At time of initial ENT review, upper aerodigestive signs/symptoms were described in 29 (53.7%) cases. Dysphagia/odynophagia was present in twenty-four (44.4%) patients, and hoarseness of voice was documented in nine (16.7%) patients. No patients were documented to have stridor on review.

Twenty-one (38.9%) patients required intubation during their admission (not including patients who were intubated, then immediately extubated for operative care). The indications for intubation were to facilitate operative intervention in nine patients, for upper airway compromise in five patients, impaired consciousness in three patients, respiratory distress in two patients, and agitation in two patients. Thirty-six (66.7%) patients required ICU admission. For patients admitted to ICU, the median length of stay was 6.5 days (IQR 3.0–14.8). The median length of hospital stay following presentation/initial suspicion of SJS/TEN was 13 (IQR 8.8–19.3) days. Six (11.1%) patients died during their admission.

Forty-one (75.9%) patients suffered oral cavity involvement, with lips being the most commonly involved subsite in thirty-three (61.1%) cases. Sixteen (29.6%) were found to have nasal cavity involvement. FNE examination found three patients (5.6%) to have nasopharyngeal mucosal involvement. Sixteen (29.6%) were documented to have oropharyngeal involvement, most commonly in the posterior pharyngeal wall (fourteen cases, 25.9%). Seventeen patients (31.5%) were identified to have laryngeal involvement, with the supraglottis most commonly implicated (sixteen cases, 29.6%). Only two cases (3.7%) had documented vocal cord involvement.

Table 1. Descriptive statistics.

Patient Demographics	Age (years)	median (IQR)	57.5 (33.5–68.3)
	Sex (male)	*n* (%)	25 (46.3%)
	Sex (female)		29 (53.7%)
SJS/TEN Factors	Total body surface area involved	median (IQR)	40.0% (30.0–70.0)
	Body surface area of desquamation		11.0% (5.0–25.8)
	SCORTEN		
	0	*n* (%)	6 (11.1%)
	1		15 (27.8%)
	2		17 (31.5%)
	3		9 (16.7%)
	4		4 (7.4%)
	≥5		3 (5.6%)
Aerodigestive Assessment Findings	Aerodigestive signs/symptoms	*n* (%)	29 (53.7%)
	Odynophagia/dysphagia		24 (44.4%)
	Hoarse voice/dysphonia		9 (16.7%)
	Stridor/shortness of breath		0 (0.0%)
	Oral cavity involvement		41 (75.9%)
	Nasal cavity involvement		16 (29.6%)
	Nasopharynx involvement		3 (5.6%)
	Oropharyngeal involvement		16 (29.6%)
	Posterior pharyngeal wall		14 (25.9%)
	Base of tongue		7 (13.0%)
	Laryngeal involvement		17 (31.5%)
	Supraglottis		16 (29.6%)
	Glottis		2 (3.7%)

No significant correlation was found between laryngeal involvement and ICU admission, intubation, or mortality on Fisher's exact test statistical analysis (Table 2). Mann–Whitney U testing demonstrated no significant difference in ICU length of stay between patients with (median 3.0 days) and without (median 3.0 days) laryngeal involvement ($U = 296$, $p = 0.7309$). Similarly, there was no significant difference in the hospital length of stay between patients with (median 12.0 days) and without (median 13.0 days) laryngeal involvement ($U = 294$, $p = 0.7084$). No significant association was established between SCORTEN and laryngeal involvement. On simple logistic regression modelling, for each increase in SCORTEN grade, the odds of laryngeal involvement were multiplied by 0.9 (95% CI 0.6–1.4).

Table 2. Subgroup analyses of laryngeal involvement vs. outcomes.

	Laryngeal Involvement *n* (%)	**No Laryngeal Involvement *n* (%)**	**Odds Ratio (95% CI)**	***p*-Value**
ICU admission	11 (64.7%)	25 (67.6%)	0.9 (0.3–3.0)	>0.9999
No ICU admission	6 (35.3%)	12 (32.4%)		
Intubation	8 (47.1%)	13 (35.1%)	1.6 (0.6–4.8)	0.5490
No intubation	9 (52.9%)	24 (64.9%)		
Mortality	2 (11.8%)	4 (10.8%)	1.1 (0.2–5.0)	>0.9999
No mortality	15 (88.2%)	33 (89.2%)		

Odds ratios were calculated via Fisher's exact test.

Simple oral cavity examination appeared to be an effective screening tool for laryngeal involvement, with oral cavity involvement of any subsite having a sensitivity of 88.2% (95% CI 65.7–97.9%) and specificity of 29.7% (95% CI 17.5–45.8%); aerodigestive signs/symptoms (odynphagia/dysphagia, hoarse voice, or stridor) had a sensitivity of 76.5% (95% CI 52.7–90.4%) and specificity of 29.7% (95% CI 17.5–45.8%) for laryngeal involvement; a combination of either oral cavity involvement or aerodigestive symptoms had a sensitivity of 94.1% (95% CI 73.0–99.7%) and specificity of 29.7% (95% CI 17.5–45.8%) for laryngeal involvement.

4. Discussion

This study represents the largest cohort of cases examining ENT manifestations of SJS/TEN in the literature [5,6,9,10]. The median age (57.5), gender (53.7% female, 46.3% male), BSA of detachment (11.0%), and total BSA involved (40.0%) were comparable to other studies [5,6,9,10]. Median SCORTEN 2 on admission and the rate of intubation (37.0%) were also similar to previously examined patient cohorts. Five patients were excluded from this review due to intubation precluding them from FNE examination. Resultantly, our study population may have lower body surface area involvement and SCORTEN by not including patients who likely had more severe disease.

Aerodigestive symptoms and signs should prompt urgent FNE to evaluate the upper airway. Despite this, we did not find any significant association between laryngeal involvement and intubation, ICU admission, or mortality. This reflects findings from similar cohorts where FNE findings were not associated with intubation [6]. Whilst this finding does not confer the risk of upper airway compromise from laryngeal involvement, it reflects that a multi-system disease such as SJS/TEN may necessitate intubation for a variety of indications. The most common reason for intubation in our cohort was to facilitate operative intervention, as patients were often subject to multiple procedures. Similarly, we did not identify statistically significant differences in length of stay in ICU or hospital for patients with laryngeal involvement. Again, considering the multi-system nature of SJS/TEN, upper aerodigestive manifestations may only represent a small part of the morbidity of this disease process. Despite no significant correlations between laryngeal involvement and ICU admission, length of stay, or intubation, the upper airway status should be considered in multidisciplinary discussions on a case-by-case basis when making decisions regarding intubation and ward or ICU disposition.

Identifying laryngeal involvement in SJS/TEN patients may confer other benefits; involvement may predict rates of pulmonary complications (including oedema, atelectasis, pneumonia), and the potential for long-term voice and swallowing impairment may be recognized [5,9]. For instance, Glasson et al. described four patients who required endoscopic surgical management of hypopharyngeal synechiae in the months following initial management of TEN [9].

FNE allows for definitive diagnosis of laryngeal involvement. Our results suggest that history and simple oral cavity examination are highly sensitive for laryngeal involvement. In our study, there was only a single case with laryngeal involvement on FNE without aerodigestive symptoms or oral cavity ulceration. The patient did not require intubation, and there was no progression of disease on serial examination. The absence of oral cavity involvement and aerodigestive signs and symptoms may reassure clinicians that laryngeal involvement is unlikely.

This study is limited by its retrospective nature. The rarity of SJS/TEN makes prospective investigation difficult. Further, a lack of standardized protocol resulted in variable time from presentation to FNE and inconsistency with repetition of FNE examination. The five patients that did not receive FNE, as they were intubated prior to ENT review, would have had a high probability of having laryngeal involvement, creating selection bias for our cohort meeting inclusion criteria. In addition, the study only observed short-term sequelae of aerodigestive SJS/TEN. Aerodigestive mucosal involvement may impact long-term voice and swallowing outcomes; this was not assessed in our study and should be addressed further in future research endeavors. Further prospective study with standardized routine nasendoscopy may provide further information of clinical progression or treatment response of aerodigestive SJS/TEN following initial diagnosis.

5. Conclusions

We did not establish a direct correlation between laryngeal involvement and clinical outcomes including intubation, ICU admission, or mortality in SJS/TEN patients. Whilst FNE remains the gold standard for diagnosing upper aerodigestive involvement, our findings suggest that history-taking and thorough oral cavity examinations are highly sensitive for detecting laryngeal involvement in patients that are not already intubated. Further research into the long-term outcomes of upper aerodigestive SJS/TEN may also help identify associated risks of chronic voice or swallow impairment.

Author Contributions: Conceptualization, M.M.X.Y. and J.P.; methodology, M.M.X.Y.; data curation, M.M.X.Y. and A.R.; writing—original draft preparation, M.M.X.Y., A.R. and M.v.A.; writing—review and editing, M.M.X.Y., A.R. and M.v.A.; supervision, J.P. All authors have read and agreed to the published version of the manuscript.

Funding: This research received no external funding.

Institutional Review Board Statement: The study was conducted in accordance with the Declaration of Helsinki, and approved by the Office of Ethics and Research Governance at Alfred Health (protocol code 674/22 and date of approval 14/12/2022).

Informed Consent Statement: Patient consent was waived in accordance with the Alfred Health Office of Ethics and Research governance policies; as this study involved previously collected clinical information, it was impracticable to obtain consent, and this project was to address internal health service provision purposes.

Data Availability Statement: The data presented in this study are available on request from the corresponding author due to the risk of patient identification in a cohort suffering a rare disease.

Acknowledgments: The authors wish to acknowledge the Ear, Nose and Throat department at Alfred Health, Victoria, Australia. This article is a revised and expanded version of a poster entitled "Retrospective Analysis of Upper Aerodigestive Manifestations of Stevens–Johnson Syndrome", which was presented at the Australian and New Zealand Burn Association Annual Scientific Meeting in Melbourne, Australia, 12–15 September 2023 [11].

Conflicts of Interest: The authors declare no conflicts of interest.

Abbreviations

The following abbreviations are used in this manuscript:

SJS	Stevens–Johnson syndrome
TEN	toxic epidermal necrolysis
SJS/TEN	Stevens–Johnson syndrome/toxic epidermal necrolysis
BSA	body surface area
FNE	flexible nasendoscopy
ICU	intensive care unit
ENT	ear, nose, and throat
SCORTEN	TEN-specific severity-of-illness score
mmol/L	millimoles per liter
CI	confidence interval

References

1. Heng, Y.; Lee, H.; Roujeau, J.C. Epidermal necrolysis: 60 years of errors and advances. *Br. J. Dermatol.* **2015**, *173*, 1250–1254. [CrossRef] [PubMed]
2. Jacobsen, A.; Olabi, B.; Langley, A.; Beecker, J.; Mutter, E.; Shelley, A.; Worley, B.; Ramsay, T.; Saavedra, A.; Parker, R. Systemic interventions for treatment of Stevens-Johnson syndrome (SJS), toxic epidermal necrolysis (TEN), and SJS/TEN overlap syndrome. *Cochrane Database Syst. Rev.* 2022. [CrossRef]
3. Frey, N.; Jossi, J.; Bodmer, M.; Bircher, A.; Jick, S.S.; Meier, C.R.; Spoendlin, J. The epidemiology of Stevens-Johnson syndrome and toxic epidermal necrolysis in the UK. *J. Investig. Dermatol.* **2017**, *137*, 1240–1247. [CrossRef] [PubMed]
4. Gibson, A.; Deshpande, P.; Campbell, C.N.; Krantz, M.S.; Mukherjee, E.; Mockenhaupt, M.; Pirmohamed, M.; Palubinsky, A.M.; Phillips, E.J. Updates on the immunopathology and genomics of severe cutaneous adverse drug reactions. *J. Allergy Clin. Immunol.* **2023**, *151*, 289–300.e284. [CrossRef] [PubMed]
5. Bequignon, E.; Duong, T.A.; Sbidian, E.; Valeyrie-Allanore, L.; Ingen-Housz-Oro, S.; Chatelin, V.; Coste, A.; Wolkenstein, P.; Chosidow, O.; Papon, J.F. Stevens-Johnson syndrome and toxic epidermal necrolysis: Ear, nose, and throat description at acute stage and after remission. *JAMA Dermatol.* **2015**, *151*, 302–307. [CrossRef] [PubMed]
6. Bhullar, H.K.; Aung, A.K.; Graudins, L.; Ihle, J.; Gin, D.; Cleland, H.; Teh, B.M. Upper airway involvement in Stevens–Johnson syndrome and toxic epidermal necrolysis. *Burns* **2020**, *46*, 682–686. [CrossRef] [PubMed]
7. Holsinger, F.C.; Kies, M.S.; Weinstock, Y.E.; Lewin, J.S.; Hajibashi, S.; Nolen, D.D.; Weber, R.; Laccourreye, O. Examination of the larynx and pharynx. *N. Engl. J. Med.* **2008**, *358*, e2. [CrossRef] [PubMed]
8. Fouchard, N.; Bertocchi, M.; Roujeau, J.-C.; Revuz, J.; Wolkenstein, P.; Bastuji-Garin, S. SCORTEN: A severity-of-illness score for toxic epidermal necrolysis. *J. Investig. Dermatol.* **2000**, *115*, 149–153. [CrossRef] [PubMed]
9. Glasson, N.; De Sandre, C.; Pantet, O.; Reinhard, A.; Lambercy, K.; Sandu, K.; Gorostidi, F. Oropharyngolaryngeal manifestations in severe toxic epidermal necrolysis: A single-center's retrospective case series. *Int. J. Dermatol.* **2023**, *62*, 1384–1390. [CrossRef] [PubMed]
10. Williams, R.; Hodge, J.; Ingram, W. Indications for intubation and early tracheostomy in patients with Stevens–Johnson syndrome and toxic epidermal necrolysis. *Am. J. Surg.* **2016**, *211*, 684–688.e681. [CrossRef] [PubMed]
11. Yii, M.; Rowson, A.; Truong, M.; Kilby, J.; Gan, C.; Prasad, J. Retrospective Analysis of Upper Aerodigestive Manifestations of Stevens-Johnson Syndrome. In Proceedings of the Australian and New Zealand Burn Association Annual Scientific Meeting, Melbourne, Australia, 12–15 September 2023.

medicina

MDPI

Article

The Modulation of Fibrosis in Vocal Fold Repair: A Study on c-Met Agonistic Antibodies and Hepatocyte Growth in Animal Studies

Hyun-Il Shin [1], Hyunsu Choi [2], Jae-Kyun Jung [3] and Choung-Soo Kim [4,*]

1 Department of Otolaryngology-Head and Neck Surgery, THANQ Seoul Thyroid-Head and Neck Surgery Center, Seoul 06912, Republic of Korea
2 Clinical Research Institute, Daejeon St. Mary's Hospital, Daejeon 34943, Republic of Korea
3 R&D Center for Innovative Medicines, Helixmith Co., Ltd., Seoul 07794, Republic of Korea
4 Department of Otolaryngology-Head and Neck Surgery, College of Medicine, The Catholic University of Korea, Seoul 06591, Republic of Korea
* Correspondence: drchoung@catholic.ac.kr; Tel.: +82-42-220-9580

Abstract: *Background and Objectives*: Damage to the vocal folds frequently results in fibrosis, which can degrade vocal quality due to the buildup of collagen and modifications in the extracellular matrix (ECM). Conventional treatments have shown limited success in reversing fibrotic changes. Hepatocyte growth factor (HGF) and c-Met-targeting antibodies are promising due to their potential to inhibit fibrosis and promote regeneration. This research examines the effectiveness of injections containing c-Met agonistic antibodies relative to HGF in reducing fibrosis within a rat model of vocal fold injury. *Materials and Methods*: Forty-five Sprague Dawley rats were divided into three groups, which were HGF, c-Met agonistic antibody, and the control (PBS). The right vocal folds were injured and treated with HGF or c-Met agonistic antibody injections. RNA isolation and quantitative real-time PCR were performed to assess mRNA levels of fibrosis-related markers at 1 and 2 weeks post-injury. Histopathological analysis was conducted at 3 weeks to evaluate collagen and hyaluronic acid (HA) deposition. *Results*: Both the HGF and c-Met groups demonstrated reduced type III collagen mRNA expression compared to the PBS group. The c-Met group uniquely maintained fibronectin levels closer to normal. Additionally, the c-Met group showed significantly upregulated expression of hyaluronan synthase (HAS) 1 and HAS 3 at 2 weeks post-injury, indicating enhanced HA synthesis. Histological analysis showed significantly lower collagen deposition and higher HA in the c-Met group than in PBS, confirming superior anti-fibrotic effects and ECM restoration. *Conclusions*: c-Met agonistic antibody injections outperformed HGF in reducing fibrosis, upregulating HAS expression, and promoting HA deposition in injured vocal folds, highlighting its potential as a superior therapeutic approach for preventing fibrosis and enhancing ECM quality in vocal fold injuries. Further research on functional outcomes in larger models is recommended to validate these findings.

Keywords: vocal fold regeneration; wound healing; scar; hepatocyte growth factor; c-Met agonistic antibody

1. Introduction

Vocal fold vibration is essential for voice production and the quality of the produced voice depends on the composition and viscoelasticity of vocal fold tissue, particularly the extracellular matrix (ECM) of the lamina propria layer. Injury to the vocal fold often leads to scar formation. This scar, along with the changes in the ECM could cause serious voice problems. Therefore, minimizing scar formation is essential during the healing process.

Vocal fold scarring is difficult to treat effectively with current surgical methods and available tissue engineering materials [1]. The lack of appropriate treatments is largely due to the limitation of existing surgical options. which do not adequately address ECM biomechanics and tissue properties. Additionally current injectable materials fail to replicate the complex structure of the ECM [2].

Numerous attempts at vocal fold regeneration have been made, including the use of mesenchymal stem cells (MSCs) [3], human nasal inferior turbinate-derived mesenchymal stem cells (hTMSCs) [4], and conditioned media [5]. However, stem cell therapy presents several challenges, like an immunological response, cost concerns, the risks of malignant transformation, etc. [6]. While therapies using conditioned media or exosome therapy could potentially overcome some limitations of stem cell therapy, identifying the most effective therapeutic components remains difficult. Hepatocyte growth factor (HGF) has also been researched as a treatment candidate for vocal fold healing due to its anti-fibrotic properties [7,8]. HGF has been shown to contribute to prevent scar formation in the liver, kidneys, and lungs in animal models [9–11]. However, a short half-time (less than five min) is the limitation of its therapeutic use [12]. The c-Met protein is a transmembrane tyrosine kinase that binds with HGF. Research has shown that c-Met localizes in endothelial cells, where the interaction between HGF and c-Met facilitates multiple biological processes [13,14].

This study investigated whether injecting a c-Met agonistic antibody, which has a relative long half-time [15], can promote the regeneration of injured vocal folds, and it compared these effects to those of HGF. We used quantitative real-time polymerase chain reaction (PCR) and histologic examination to analyze the early phase of wound healing in rat vocal fold injury models [5].

2. Materials and Methods

2.1. Animal Experiments

Approval for this study was granted by the Animal Ethics Committee of the Catholic University of Korea (permit no. CMCDJ-AP-2022-001), and all procedures followed institutional care guidelines. Forty-five Sprague Dawley rats were divided among three groups, with 12 each in the HGF and c-Met experimental groups and 12 in the PBS control group, with three animals from each group reserved for histological analysis. The animals were anesthetized with ketamine hydrochloride (100 mg/kg) and xylazine hydrochloride (10 mg/kg), positioned semi-vertically on a custom platform and visualized using a pediatric endoscope. Microscissors were used to expose the thyroarytenoid muscle on the right vocal folds, while the left vocal fold served as an untreated control. Immediately following injury, 100 ng of HGF (Millipore, Bedford, MA, USA) in 50 μL PBS or 100 ng of c-Met agonistic antibody (Helixmith, Seoul, Republic of Korea) in 50 μL PBS was injected into the injury site for experimental groups. The PBS control group received an injection of 50 μL PBS alone. All injections were administered under direct visualization using a 30-gauge needle and pediatric laryngoscope.

2.2. RNA Isolation and Real-Time PCR of Rat Vocal Fold Tissues

The rat vocal folds were collected at 1 and 2 weeks post-injury and homogenized using a TissueLyser II (Qiagen, Valencia, CA, USA). RNA extraction was carried out with TRIzol reagent (Invitrogen, Carlsbad, CA, USA), then ribonuclease-free deoxyribonuclease I (Qiagen) was used to minimize contamination from genomic DNA. Complementary DNA (cDNA) was synthesized using a Reverse Transcriptase Premix Kit (Elpis Biotech, Daejeon, Republic of Korea) with 1 μg of RNA. Real-time PCR was conducted on an ABI 7500 FAST system (Applied Biosystems, Foster City, CA, USA) in a 20 μL reaction volume, containing Power SYBR Green PCR Master Mix (Applied Biosystems), 500 nM forward and reverse primers, and 1 μL of cDNA. mRNA expression levels were normalized against glyceraldehyde-3-phosphate dehydrogenase (GAPDH).

Primer sets used in this study are shown in Table 1.

Table 1. Primer information.

	Sequence	
Rat Genes	**Forward**	**Reverse**
GAPDH	5′-ACCACAGTCCATGCCATCAC-3′	5′-TCCACCACCCTGTTGCTGTA-3′
COL III	5′-CACTGGGGAATGGAGCAAAAC-3′	5′-ATCAGGACCACCAATGTCATAGG-3′
FN	5′-CGAGGTGACAGAGACCACAA-3′	5′-CTGGAGTCAAGCCAGACACA-3′
HAS 1	5′-TAGGTGCTGTTGGAGGAGATGTGA-3′	5′-AAGCTCGCTCCACATTGAAGGCTA-3′
HAS 2	5′-CCAATGCAGTTTCGGTGATG-3′	5′-ACTTGGACCGAGCCGTGTAT-3′
HAS 3	5′-CCTCATCGCCACAGTCATACAA-3′	5′-CCACCAGCTGCACCGTTAG-3′
MMP2	5′-GTCACTCCGCTGCGCTTTTCTCG-3′	5′-GACACATGGGGCACCTTCTGA-3′

Abbreviations: *GAPDH*, glyceraldehyde-3-phosphate dehydrogenase; *COL III*, collagen type III; *FN*, fibronectin; *HAS*, hyaluronan synthase; *MMP2*, Matrix metalloproteinase-2.

2.3. Histopathological Analysis of Rat Vocal Fold Tissue

Three larynges from each group were collected for histological examination following euthanasia, three weeks after injury. The tissues were embedded in paraffin, sectioned coronally at a thickness of 4 µm using a microtome, and stained with hematoxylin and eosin. Verhoeff–Van Gieson and Masson's trichrome were used for the detection of collagen fiber and elastic fiber, following standard pathology protocols. Prepared slides were examined under a light microscope (Eclipse TE300; Nikon, Tokyo, Japan). Densitometric analysis was conducted to quantify extracellular matrix staining, with areas measured using ImageJ software (Version 1.53e, National Institutes of Health, Bethesda, MD, USA).

2.4. Statistics

Results are presented as means with standard error of the mean (SEM). GraphPad Prism 5 (GraphPad, Inc., La Jolla, CA, USA) was used for conducting statistical analyses. To compare multiple groups, a one-way ANOVA was followed by Tukey's post hoc test. A p-value of less than 0.05 was used to determine statistical significance.

3. Results

3.1. Gene Expression at 1 Week Post-Injury

The expression levels of mRNAs encoding hyaluronan synthase (HAS) 1, HAS 2, and HAS 3 did not differ among the normal, PBS, HGF, and c-Met groups. The mRNA expression level of procollagen type III (COL III) was significantly downregulated in both the c-Met and HGF groups compared with the PBS group, while the gene encoding fibronectin (FN) was upregulated in the PBS and HGF groups compared with the normal group. However, in the c-Met group, the mRNA level of FN expression did not increase as much as in the PBS and HGF groups, showing no significant difference compared to the normal group (Figure 1).

3.2. Gene Expression at 2 Weeks Post-Injury

At two weeks post-injury, the mRNA expression levels of HAS 1 and HAS 3 were significantly upregulated in the c-Met group compared to the normal group. HAS 2 expression in the c-Met group showed an increasing trend, although it did not reach statistical significance. In the HGF group, only HAS 3 mRNA expression was significantly upregulated compared to the normal group. COL III mRNA expression was significantly upregulated in the PBS group compared to the normal group and was significantly downregulated in both the HGF and c-Met groups. FN was upregulated in the PBS, HGF, and c-Met groups compared with the normal group, but FN was downregulated in the c-Met group compared to the PBS group (Figure 2).

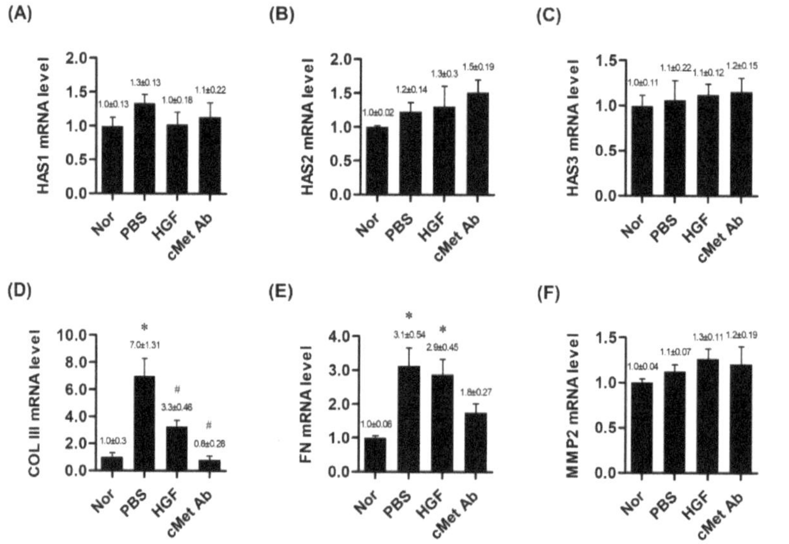

Figure 1. mRNA expression ratios of genes related to vocal fold tissue regeneration in the normal, PBS, and c-Met Ab groups on post-injury day 7. * $p < 0.05$ vs. Nor (normal), # $p < 0.05$ vs. PBS, $p < 0.05$ vs. HGF. (**A–C**) Expression levels of HAS1, HAS2, and HAS3 mRNA, respectively. (**D**) mRNA expression of COL III. (**E**) mRNA expression of FN. (**F**) mRNA expression of MMP2. Normal (Nor) tissues were compared to injured tissues treated with phosphate-buffered saline (PBS), hepatocyte growth factor (HGF), or c-Met agonistic antibody (c-Met Ab).

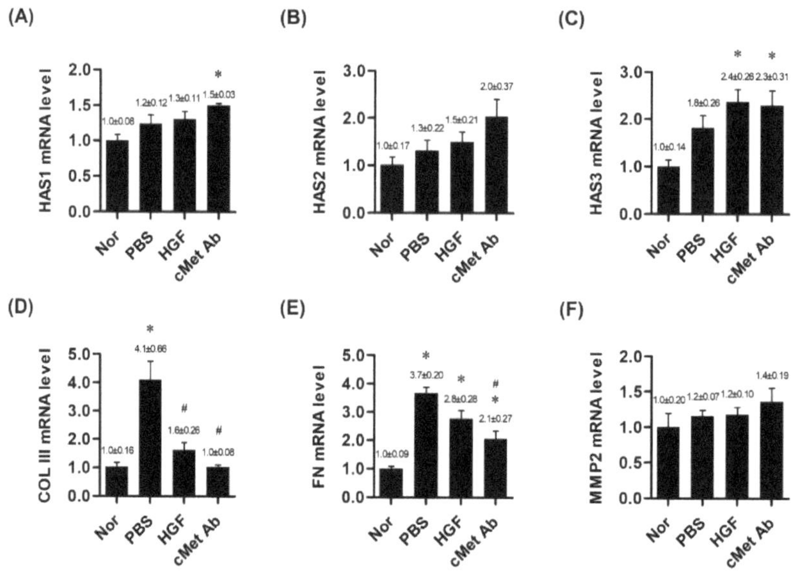

Figure 2. mRNA expression ratios of genes related to vocal fold tissue regeneration in the normal, PBS, and c-Met Ab groups on post-injury day 14. * $p < 0.05$ vs. Nor (normal), # $p < 0.05$ vs. PBS, $p < 0.05$ vs. HGF. (**A–C**) Expression levels of HAS1, HAS2, and HAS3 mRNA, respectively. (**D**) mRNA expression of COL III. (**E**) mRNA expression of FN. (**F**) mRNA expression of MMP2. Normal (Nor) tissues were compared to injured tissues treated with phosphate-buffered saline (PBS), hepatocyte growth factor (HGF), or c-Met agonistic antibody (c-Met Ab).

3.3. Histological Examination

Histological analysis was conducted at 3 weeks post-injury. A densitometric analysis of histological samples showed that the c-Met groups exhibited stronger anti-fibrotic effects than the PBS group. Masson's trichrome staining indicated significantly reduced collagen deposition in the c-Met groups compared to the PBS group. Although the HGF group also showed reduced collagen deposition compared to the PBS group, the difference was not statistically significant. HA was detected by alcian blue staining. The c-Met group exhibited significantly increased HA deposition compared to the PBS group. The HGF group also showed increased HA deposition compared to the PBS group, though this difference did not reach statistical significance (Figure 3).

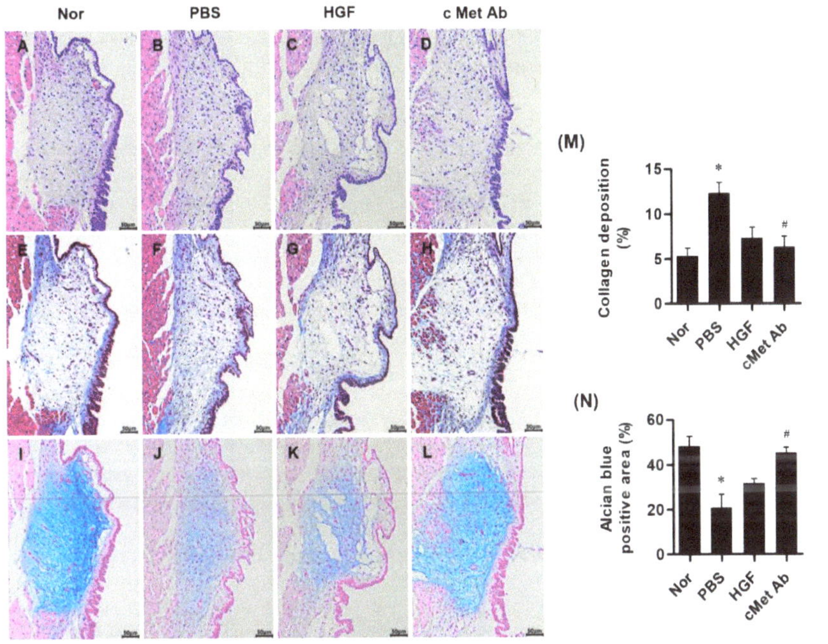

Figure 3. Representative images of stained vocal fold tissues at 3 weeks post-injury: hematoxylin and eosin staining (**A–D**), Masson's trichrome staining for collagen (**E–H**), and alcian blue staining for hyaluronic acid (**I–L**) from the normal (Nor), PBS, HGF, and c-Met Ab groups. Scale bars = 50 μm. Quantitative analysis of collagen deposition (blue-stained collagen) (**M**) and alcian blue-positive area (blue-colored hyaluronic acids) (**N**) are shown. Original magnification: 200×; * $p < 0.05$ compared to Nor (normal), # $p < 0.05$ compared to PBS, and $p < 0.05$ compared to HGF.

4. Discussion

Scarring after vocal fold injuries is a prevalent cause of severe voice impairment. The scarring process includes three main phases, namely the inflammatory response, cellular proliferation, and tissue remodeling [16].

Inflammatory factors are produced within 4 to 8 h post-injury, after which there is an upregulation of hyaluronan synthases I and II and procollagens I and III, followed by a substantial recruitment of cells, mainly with fibroblastic characteristics, originating from the macula flava. On days 5–7 post-injury, the fibroblasts undergo differentiation myofibroblasts, leading to a disorganization of collagen and elastin bundles and a reduction in the density of elastin and hyaluronic acid. Subsequently, type III collagen is replaced by type I collagen, and the density of fibronectin increases [17,18]. Vocal fold scarring is characterized by excessive collagen deposition. Thus, reducing collagen production is crucial to decreasing scar formation. While fibronectin is necessary for wound healing, prolonged upregulated fibronectin expression after injury causes fibrosis and impairs the viscoelastic properties of the vocal fold [19]. The key component of vocal fold viscoelastic properties is hyaluronic acid; therefore, HA synthesis is important [20,21]. HAS genes have three subtypes, with HAS2 and HAS3 exhibiting higher enzymatic activity compared to HAS1 [22].

The key focus in the wound healing process is to reduce scarring and restore the normal composition of the lamina propria, which is distinct from simply accelerating wound closure. A recent study, although conducted on skin tissue, reported that blocking potassium channels promotes wound healing [23]. However, this study did not include histological analysis, making it difficult to determine the extent of scar formation compared to normal tissue. The researchers hypothesized that fibroblast migration and activation at the wound site accelerate wound healing. However, based on previous studies, such mechanisms are known to potentially exacerbate scarring [24,25].

In this study, both the c-Met and HGF groups exhibited reduced COL III mRNA expression at 1 or 2 weeks post-injury. However, in the c-Met group, FN mRNA expression did not increase relative to the normal group at 1 week post-injury and decreased compared to the PBS group at 2 weeks post-injury. Regarding HA, no differences were observed in the RNA expression levels of HAS1, HAS2, or HAS3 at 1 week post-injury. However, by 2 weeks post-injury, a significant increase in HAS3 mRNA expression was detected. This finding aligns with previous studies, which report an initial rise in HAS1 and HAS2—especially HAS2—within three days post-injury, followed by a subsequent increase in HAS3 [26]. Furthermore, the observed significant upregulation of HAS3 mRNA expression in both the HGF and c-Met groups is consistent with earlier research suggesting that HGF negatively regulates TGF-β, which is known to suppress HAS3 expression during tissue injury. After 3 weeks, the histologic examination confirmed that mRNA expression correlated with histological change. The c-Met group had less collagen and more HA deposition, demonstrating a more pronounced anti-fibrotic effect than the PBS group with significance. However, there was no statistical difference from the HGF group. In this report, we demonstrated that the c-Met antagonistic antibody performs better than the HGF and PBS group in the anti-fibrotic effects of vocal fold injury.

Currently used injectable materials for the vocal folds primarily aim to improve glottic closure, with Radiesse (Merz North America, Inc., Raleigh, NC, USA) providing long-term effects and hyaluronic acid (HA) offering short-term effects [27,28]. These materials are typically injected either into or outside the thyroarytenoid muscle to facilitate vocal fold adduction with a space-occupying effect [29]. However, their purpose differs from regenerating the lamina propria during the wound healing process of vocal fold injuries

The restoration of normal vocal fold properties is essential to the treatment of vocal fold scars.

Many attempts have been made to reduce vocal fold fibrosis following injury.

In tissue engineering, the regeneration of tissues or organs can be achieved by the combination of scaffolds, cells, and regulators under proper conditions. Growth factor therapy is one of the therapeutic strategies in regenerative medicine. Multiple studies have highlighted HGF's efficacy as a promising growth factor therapy for vocal fold scarring, demonstrating its capacity to regulate ECM production in fibroblasts [7,14,30,31].

In vocal fold regeneration, HGF and c-Met expression, known for their anti-fibrotic effects, decrease immediately following vocal fold injury but increase again after 14 days [32]. This period is considered critical for vocal fold scar remodeling. Supplementing the diminished HGF effect, such as through external administration, may aid in preventing scar formation in the vocal folds [30,32]. However, the effectiveness of HGF might be limited by its short half-life, necessitating repeated injection or the use of slow-release scaffolds [33–35].

Repeated injections may damage the vocal folds, potentially hindering the healing process [36]. Slow-release scaffolds, although designed for sustained release, do not replicate the precise biomechanical properties of the native ECM, which may interfere with vocal fold vibration until fully degraded [29,37]. Additionally, scaffold degradation may trigger inflammatory responses, posing further risks [38]. Therefore, a single, long-acting injection without a scaffold would be more suitable for effective treatment. The c-Met agonistic antibody is administered in a single injection with PBS, eliminating the need for scaffold use.

Recently, studies have explored the use of HGF-transfected stem cells via viral vectors to extend the effects of HGF [39]. However, the use of stem cells poses challenges, such as immunological responses and the risk of malignant transformation, as previously noted. While autologous or homologous stem cells may reduce these risks, they present issues related to consistency and cost. Additionally, viral transfection techniques are limited by concerns over mutations and stability [40,41]. In contrast, the c-Met agonistic antibody offers a cell-free, virus-free therapeutic approach, potentially circumventing these issues.

The serum half-life of the c-Met agonistic antibody used in this study had a half-life of approximately 3 days, with persistence in the body for up to 6 days following intravenous injection [15]. Therefore, this agonistic antibody has the potential to compensate for the short half-life of HGF.

In this report, we demonstrated that the c-Met antagonistic antibody performs better than the HGF and PBS group in anti-fibrotic effects during the remodeling of injured vocal folds. However, there were some limitations; first, while the c-Met group was more effective in anti-fibrosis than the HGF group, the difference was smaller than expected. To clarify this daily examination of the activated c-Met receptor, mRNA expression of CoLIII, FN, and HAS following injection may be beneficial. Additionally, conducting histological examinations beyond three weeks post-injury would further enhance our understanding of the findings. But conducting such experiments would require a significantly larger number of experimental animals compared to the current study. Second, the regeneration of vocal fold tissue does not necessarily guarantee functional restoration of vocal fold abilities. Therefore, to evaluate the function of the recovered vocal folds (such as the symmetrical mucosa waves during phonation between control and study group vocal folds), additional experiments involving larger animal models, such as rabbits, and tools like high-speed video cameras are required. If additional experiments are conducted considering these limitations, it is believed that the c-Met agonist antibody can be used in human research.

5. Conclusions

The injection of a c-Met agonistic antibody into injured vocal folds showed an anti-fibrotic effect in the early phase of wound healing, demonstrating superiority over HGF injection. These findings highlight the potential of c-Met agonistic antibodies for regenerative therapy in vocal fold injuries.

Author Contributions: C.-S.K. designed the study. H.C. analyzed and interpreted the data. J.-K.J. provided technical support and the c-Met antibody. C.-S.K. and H.C. conducted the experiments. C.-S.K. and H.-I.S. prepared the manuscript. H.-I.S. reviewed and edited the manuscript. All authors have read and agreed to the published version of the manuscript.

Funding: This work was supported by a Clinical Research Institute grant funded by The Catholic University of Korea Daejeon St. Mary's Hospital (CMCDJ-P-2023-001) and The E.N.T. Fund of the Catholic University of Korea made in the program year of 2023.

Institutional Review Board Statement: The study was approved by the Animal Ethics Committee of the Catholic University of Korea (permit no. CMCDJ-AP-2022-001). Approval date: 24 June 2022.

Informed Consent Statement: Not applicable.

Data Availability Statement: The datasets generated during and/or analyzed during the current study are available from the corresponding author on reasonable request.

Acknowledgments: Helixmith Co., Ltd., Seoul, Republic of Korea, provided the c-Met-agonistic antibody (c-Met Ab (VM507)) for the experiments. Choung-Soo Kim wishes to acknowledge the financial support of the Catholic Medical Center Research Foundation made in the program year of 2023.

Conflicts of Interest: Author Jae-Kyun Jung was employed by the company Helixmith Co., Ltd. The remaining authors declare that the research was conducted in the absence of any commercial or financial relationships that could be construed as a potential conflict of interest.

Abbreviations

List of abbreviations used in this manuscript.

Abbreviations	Definition
ECM	Extracellular matrix
HGF	Hepatocyte growth factor
PBS	Phosphate buffered saline
RNA	Ribonucleic Acid
HA	Hyaluronic acid
HAS	Hyaluronan synthase
MSC	Mesenchymal stem cells
PCR	Polymerase chain reaction
DNA	Deoxyribonucleic acid
COLIII	Procollagen type III
FN	Fibronectin
TGF-β	Transforming growth factors-beta superfamily

References

1. Thibeault, S.L.; Klemuk, S.A.; Chen, X.; Quinchia Johnson, B.H. In Vivo engineering of the vocal fold ECM with injectable HA hydrogels-late effects on tissue repair and biomechanics in a rabbit model. *J. Voice* **2011**, *25*, 249–253. [CrossRef] [PubMed]
2. Nagubothu, S.R.; Sugars, R.V.; Tudzarovski, N.; Andrén, A.T.; Bottai, M.; Davies, L.C.; Hertegård, S.; Le Blanc, K. Mesenchymal stromal cells modulate tissue repair responses within the injured vocal fold. *Laryngoscope* **2020**, *130*, E21–E29. [CrossRef] [PubMed]
3. Cedervall, J.; Ahrlund-Richter, L.; Svensson, B.; Forsgren, K.; Maurer, F.H.; Vidovska, D.; Hertegård, S. Injection of embryonic stem cells into scarred rabbit vocal folds enhances healing and improves viscoelasticity: Short-term results. *Laryngoscope* **2007**, *117*, 2075–2081. [CrossRef] [PubMed]
4. Kim, C.S.; Choi, H.; Park, K.C.; Kim, S.W.; Sun, D.I. The Ability of Human Nasal Inferior Turbinate-Derived Mesenchymal Stem Cells to Repair Vocal Fold Injuries. *Otolaryngol. Head Neck Surg.* **2018**, *159*, 335–342. [CrossRef]
5. Kim, C.S.; Choi, H.; Kim, S.W.; Sun, D.I. The Ability of Conditioned Media from Stem Cells to Repair Vocal Fold Injuries. *Laryngoscope* **2019**, *129*, 1867–1875. [CrossRef]
6. Baglio, S.R.; Pegtel, D.M.; Baldini, N. Mesenchymal stem cell secreted vesicles provide novel opportunities in (stem) cell-free therapy. *Front. Physiol.* **2012**, *3*, 359. [CrossRef]
7. Kishimoto, Y.; Hirano, S.; Suehiro, A.; Tateya, I.; Kanemaru, S.; Nakamura, T.; Ito, J. Effect of exogenous hepatocyte growth factor on vocal fold fibroblasts. *Ann. Otol. Rhinol. Laryngol.* **2009**, *118*, 606–611. [CrossRef]
8. Choi, J.S.; Heang Oh, S.; Kim, Y.M.; Lim, J.Y. Hyaluronic Acid/Alginate Hydrogel Containing Hepatocyte Growth Factor and Promotion of Vocal Fold Wound Healing. *Tissue Eng. Regen. Med.* **2020**, *17*, 651–658. [CrossRef]
9. Schievenbusch, S.; Strack, I.; Scheffler, M.; Wennhold, K.; Maurer, J.; Nischt, R.; Dienes, H.P.; Odenthal, M. Profiling of anti-fibrotic signaling by hepatocyte growth factor in renal fibroblasts. *Biochem. Biophys. Res. Commun.* **2009**, *385*, 55–61. [CrossRef]
10. Chakraborty, S.; Chopra, P.; Hak, A.; Dastidar, S.G.; Ray, A. Hepatocyte growth factor is an attractive target for the treatment of pulmonary fibrosis. *Expert Opin. Investig. Drugs* **2013**, *22*, 499–515. [CrossRef]
11. Ishikawa, H.; Jo, J.; Tabata, Y. Liver Anti-Fibrosis Therapy with Mesenchymal Stem Cells Secreting Hepatocyte Growth Factor. *J. Biomater. Sci. Polym. Ed.* **2012**, *23*, 2259–2272. [CrossRef] [PubMed]
12. Moreno, E.; Meneu, J.C.; Calvo, J.; Pérez, B.; Sesma, A.G.; Manrique, A.; Vegh, I.; Aragón, A.M.; Grau, M.; Gimeno, A.; et al. Modulation of hepatocyte growth factor plasma levels in relation to the dose of exogenous heparin administered: An experimental study in rats. *Transplant. Proc.* **2005**, *37*, 3943–3947. [CrossRef] [PubMed]
13. Zhang, Y.; Xia, M.; Jin, K.; Wang, S.; Wei, H.; Fan, C.; Wu, Y.; Li, X.; Li, X.; Li, G.; et al. Function of the c-Met receptor tyrosine kinase in carcinogenesis and associated therapeutic opportunities. *Mol. Cancer* **2018**, *17*, 45. [CrossRef] [PubMed]
14. Hirano, S.; Thibeault, S.; Bless, D.M.; Ford, C.N.; Kanemaru, S. Hepatocyte growth factor and its receptor c-met in rat and rabbit vocal folds. *Ann. Otol. Rhinol. Laryngol.* **2002**, *111*, 661–666. [CrossRef]
15. An, J.N.; Li, L.; Lee, J.; Yu, S.S.; Lee, J.; Kim, Y.C.; Kim, D.K.; Oh, Y.K.; Lim, C.S.; Kim, Y.S.; et al. cMet agonistic antibody attenuates apoptosis in ischaemia-reperfusion-induced kidney injury. *J. Cell. Mol. Med.* **2020**, *24*, 5640–5651. [CrossRef]
16. Schultz, G.S.; Chin, G.A.; Moldawer, L.; Diegelmann, R.F. Principles of wound healing. In *Mechanisms of Vascular Disease: A Reference Book for Vascular Specialists [Internet]*; University of Adelaide Press: Adelaide, Australia, 2011.
17. Singh, D.; Rai, V.; Agrawal, D.K. Regulation of Collagen I and Collagen III in Tissue Injury and Regeneration. *Cardiol. Cardiovasc. Med.* **2023**, *7*, 5–16. [CrossRef]

18. Mattei, A.; Magalon, J.; Bertrand, B.; Philandrianos, C.; Veran, J.; Giovanni, A. Cell therapy and vocal fold scarring. *Eur. Ann. Otorhinolaryngol. Head Neck Dis.* **2017**, *134*, 339–345. [CrossRef]
19. Rousseau, B.; Ge, P.J.; Ohno, T.; French, L.C.; Thibeault, S.L. Extracellular matrix gene expression after vocal fold injury in a rabbit model. *Ann. Otol. Rhinol. Laryngol.* **2008**, *117*, 598–603. [CrossRef]
20. Kazemirad, S.; Heris, H.K.; Mongeau, L. Viscoelasticity of hyaluronic acid-gelatin hydrogels for vocal fold tissue engineering. *J. Biomed. Mater. Res. B Appl. Biomater.* **2016**, *104*, 283–290. [CrossRef]
21. Walimbe, T.; Panitch, A.; Sivasankar, P.M. A Review of Hyaluronic Acid and Hyaluronic Acid-based Hydrogels for Vocal Fold Tissue Engineering. *J. Voice* **2017**, *31*, 416–423. [CrossRef]
22. Siiskonen, H.; Oikari, S.; Pasonen-Seppänen, S.; Rilla, K. Hyaluronan synthase 1: A mysterious enzyme with unexpected functions. *Front. Immunol.* **2015**, *6*, 43. [CrossRef] [PubMed]
23. Grigore, A.; Vatasescu-Balcan, A.; Stoleru, S.; Zugravu, A.; Poenaru, E.; Engi, M.; Coman, O.A.; Fulga, I. Experimental Research on the Influence of Ion Channels on the Healing of Skin Wounds in Rats. *Processes* **2024**, *12*, 109. [CrossRef]
24. McDougall, S.; Dallon, J.; Sherratt, J.; Maini, P. Fibroblast migration and collagen deposition during dermal wound healing: Mathematical modelling and clinical implications. *Philos. Trans. A Math. Phys. Eng. Sci.* **2006**, *364*, 1385–1405. [CrossRef] [PubMed]
25. Shin, D.; Minn, K.W. The effect of myofibroblast on contracture of hypertrophic scar. *Plast. Reconstr. Surg.* **2004**, *113*, 633–640. [CrossRef] [PubMed]
26. Bai, K.J.; Spicer, A.P.; Mascarenhas, M.M.; Yu, L.; Ochoa, C.D.; Garg, H.G.; Quinn, D.A. The role of hyaluronan synthase 3 in ventilator-induced lung injury. *Am. J. Respir. Crit. Care Med.* **2005**, *172*, 92–98. [CrossRef]
27. Halderman, A.A.; Bryson, P.C.; Benninger, M.S.; Chota, R. Safety and length of benefit of restylane for office-based injection medialization-a retrospective review of one institution's experience. *J. Voice* **2014**, *28*, 631–635. [CrossRef]
28. Kwon, T.K.; Lee, J.E.; Cha, W.J.; Song, C.M.; Sung, M.W.; Kim, K.H. Serial computed tomographic and positron emission tomographic properties of injection material used for vocal fold augmentation. *Laryngoscope* **2013**, *123*, 2491–2496. [CrossRef]
29. Kwon, S.; Choi, H.; Park, C.; Choi, S.; Kim, E.; Kim, S.W.; Kim, C.-S.; Koo, H. In vivo vocal fold augmentation using an injectable polyethylene glycol hydrogel based on click chemistry. *Biomater. Sci.* **2021**, *9*, 108–115. [CrossRef]
30. Chen, H.; Erndt-Marino, J.; Diaz-Rodriguez, P.; Kulwatno, J.; Jimenez-Vergara, A.C.; Thibeault, S.L.; Hahn, M.S. In vitro evaluation of anti-fibrotic effects of select cytokines for vocal fold scar treatment. *J. Biomed. Mater. Res. B Appl. Biomater.* **2019**, *107*, 1056–1067. [CrossRef]
31. Dias Garcia, R.I.; Tsuji, D.H.; Imamura, R.; Mauad, T.; Ferraz da Silva, L.F. Effects of hepatocyte growth factor injection and reinjection on healing in the rabbit vocal fold. *J. Voice* **2012**, *26*, 667.e7–667.e12. [CrossRef]
32. Xu, H.; Fan, G.K. The Role of Cytokines in Modulating Vocal Fold Fibrosis: A Contemporary Review. *Laryngoscope* **2021**, *131*, 139–145. [CrossRef] [PubMed]
33. Mizuta, M.; Hirano, S.; Kishimoto, Y.; Hiwatashi, N.; Tateya, I.; Kanemaru, S.; Nakamura, T.; Ito, J. Pharmacokinetics and safety of human recombinant hepatocyte growth factor administered to vocal folds. *Laryngoscope* **2014**, *124*, 2131–2135. [CrossRef] [PubMed]
34. Choi, J.S.; Lee, S.; Kim, D.Y.; Kim, Y.M.; Kim, M.S.; Lim, J.Y. Functional remodeling after vocal fold injury by small intestinal submucosa gel containing hepatocyte growth factor. *Biomaterials* **2015**, *40*, 98–106. [CrossRef] [PubMed]
35. Choi, Y.H.; Ahn, H.J.; Park, M.R.; Han, M.J.; Lee, J.H.; Kwon, S.K. Dual growth factor-immobilized bioactive injection material for enhanced treatment of glottal insufficiency. *Acta Biomater.* **2019**, *86*, 269–279. [CrossRef]
36. Shi, L.L.; Giraldez-Rodriguez, L.A.; Johns, M.M., 3rd. The Risk of Vocal Fold Atrophy after Serial Corticosteroid Injections of the Vocal Fold. *J. Voice* **2016**, *30*, 762.e11–762.e13. [CrossRef]
37. Klemuk, S.A.; Titze, I.R. Viscoelastic properties of three vocal-fold injectable biomaterials at low audio frequencies. *Laryngoscope* **2004**, *114*, 1597–1603. [CrossRef]
38. Li, L.; Stiadle, J.M.; Lau, H.K.; Zerdoum, A.B.; Jia, X.; Thibeault, S.L.; Kiick, K.L. Tissue engineering-based therapeutic strategies for vocal fold repair and regeneration. *Biomaterials* **2016**, *108*, 91–110. [CrossRef]
39. Xie, X.; Li, X.; Lin, X.; Chen, X.; Zhang, C.; Sun, G. Effects of hepatocyte growth factor-transfected mesenchymal stem cell transplantation in canine injured vocal folds. *Growth Factors* **2023**, *41*, 130–139. [CrossRef]
40. Fang, Y.; Gong, X.; Xu, M.; Zeng, F.; Zhang, J. A self-deletion lentiviral vector to reduce the risk of replication-competent virus formation. *J. Gene Med.* **2013**, *15*, 102–112. [CrossRef]
41. Schambach, A.; Zychlinski, D.; Ehrnstroem, B.; Baum, C. Biosafety features of lentiviral vectors. *Hum. Gene Ther.* **2013**, *24*, 132–142. [CrossRef]

medicina

MDPI

Article

Real-World Evaluation of Dupilumab in the Long-Term Management of Eosinophilic Chronic Rhinosinusitis with Nasal Polyps: A Focus on IL-4 and IL-13 Receptor Blockade

Nicola Lombardo [1,*], Aurelio D'Ecclesia [2], Emanuela Chiarella [3], Corrado Pelaia [4], Debbie Riccelli [1], Annamaria Ruzza [2], Nadia Lobello [1,†] and Giovanna Lucia Piazzetta [1,†]

1 Otolaryngology Head and Neck Surgery, Department Medical and Surgical Sciences, University "Magna Graecia" of Catanzaro, 88100 Catanzaro, Italy; debbie.riccelli001@studenti.unicz.it (D.R.); nadialobello@gmail.com (N.L.); giovannapiazzetta@hotmail.it (G.L.P.)
2 Department of Maxillofacial Surgery and Otolaryngology, IRCCS Casa Sollievo della Sofferenza, 71013 Foggia, Italy; aureliodecclesia73@gmail.com (A.D.); ruzza_annamaria@libero.it (A.R.)
3 Laboratory of Molecular Haematopoiesis and Stem Cell Biology, Department of Experimental and Clinical Medicine, University "Magna Graecia" of Catanzaro, 88100 Catanzaro, Italy; emanuelachiarella@unicz.it
4 Department of Health Sciences, University "Magna Graecia" of Catanzaro, 88100 Catanzaro, Italy; pelaia.corrado@gmail.com
* Correspondence: nlombardo@unicz.it; Tel.: +39-331-380-3904
† These authors contributed equally to this work.

Abstract: *Background and Objectives*: Chronic rhinosinusitis (CRS) is a complex inflammatory condition of the nasal passages that severely impairs quality of life. Type 2 CRS is characterized by eosinophilic inflammation, driven by cytokines like IL-4, IL-5, and IL-13. These cytokines are key to CRS pathogenesis and contribute to a heavy disease burden, especially with comorbidities. This study assessed dupilumab, a monoclonal antibody targeting IL-4 and IL-13 signaling, to evaluate its efficacy in reducing the disease burden in patients with CRS with nasal polyps (CRSwNP). *Materials and Methods*: The patients received subcutaneous dupilumab for 42 weeks. The outcomes included Nasal Polyp Score (NPS); Sino-Nasal Outcome Test (SNOT-22), Numeric Rating Scale (NRS), and Visual Analog Scale (VAS) scores; total IgE; and olfactory function. *Results*: Significant improvements were observed across the NPS and SNOT-22, NRS, and VAS scores after 42 weeks. Their total IgE levels were reduced, though a transient increase in peripheral eosinophilia appeared at 16 weeks. The patients also reported substantial improvements in olfactory function and high satisfaction with the treatment, supporting dupilumab's potential in reducing both symptom severity and inflammation in CRSwNP. *Conclusions*: These results indicate that dupilumab may be an effective treatment for CRSwNP, offering significant symptom relief, improved olfactory function, and enhanced quality of life. High satisfaction levels suggest that dupilumab may provide therapeutic advantages over the conventional CRS treatments, though further studies are warranted to confirm its long-term benefits.

Keywords: chronic rhinosinusitis; nasal polyps; dupilumab; type 2 inflammation; non-type 2 inflammation

1. Introduction

Chronic rhinosinusitis (CRS) is a multifaceted inflammatory condition that affects both the nasal mucosa and paranasal sinuses.

It presents as two main phenotypes: chronic rhinosinusitis without nasal polyps (CRSsNP) and chronic rhinosinusitis with nasal polyps (CRSwNP). CRSwNP, often associated with more severe symptoms and comorbid conditions like asthma, can be further classified based on the inflammatory pathways—most notably type 2 inflammation, which is characterized by eosinophilic activity and elevated levels of cytokines such as IL-4, IL-5, and IL-13. This type of inflammation plays a significant role in refractory CRS cases, where the traditional treatments often fail to provide long-term relief [1–3].

Management of CRS has historically relied on corticosteroids and surgery, but these interventions often fall short, particularly in patients with severe or recurrent CRSwNP. In recent years, a better understanding of the immunological mechanisms driving CRS has led to the development of biologic therapies.

Recently, a population of mesenchymal stem cells (MSCs) was also identified in nasal polyps, which may be implicated in the inflammation process considering their immunomodulatory properties. However, the MSCs' contribution to the microenvironment of nasal polyps still needs to be clarified [4–7]. The two types of inflammation are often age-related: in the elderly, there is less eosinophilic infiltration, which is known to increase the risk of recurrence [8,9].

Similarly, among young patients, there is a significantly higher prevalence of allergies. These data suggest that when CRS appears in the elderly, the pathogenesis is different and less linked to allergy and eosinophilic infiltration but more to the formation of nasal polyps [10].

Biologics offer a more targeted approach by blocking specific cytokines and immune pathways involved in type 2 inflammation. These therapies have transformed the treatment landscape for patients with severe CRSwNP who are unresponsive to the conventional treatments. Biologics such as omalizumab (anti-IgE), mepolizumab and reslizumab (anti-IL-5), and dupilumab (anti-IL-4/IL-13) have shown significant efficacy in reducing polyp size, improving symptoms, and reducing the need for corticosteroids or surgery. Dupilumab in particular has become the first monoclonal antibody approved for treating CRSwNP, demonstrating strong efficacy in clinical trials. These biologic therapies not only address the underlying inflammation but also improve the quality of life of patients, reducing the frequency of symptom recurrence and the need for invasive procedures [11–14].

In this study, we present findings from administering dupilumab to a cohort of 40 CRSwNP patients, focusing on its impact on key clinical parameters such as symptom scores, polyp size, and biomarkers like total IgE and peripheral eosinophilia.

2. Materials and Methods

2.1. Study Design

This study was a single-arm, pre-post-interventional study conducted across multiple centers. It evaluated the effects of subcutaneous dupilumab administration over 42 weeks in patients with chronic rhinosinusitis with nasal polyps (CRSwNP). No randomization or control group was included in this design. Clinical outcomes, such as the Nasal Polyp Score (NPS) and SNOT-22, were measured at baseline and after 42 weeks of treatment to assess the intervention's effectiveness.

This study was conducted at multiple centers, following ethical guidelines as stipulated in the Declaration of Helsinki. The study protocol received approval from the institutional review boards of each participating site, and all of the participants provided written informed consent prior to enrollment.

2.2. The Nasal Polyp Score (NPS)

To assess the Nasal Polyp Score (NPS), nasal endoscopy was performed using an OLYMPUS ENF TYPE-GP fiberscope. This procedure was conducted across multiple centers, including the ENT Department of the University Hospital "Mater Domini" in Catanzaro and the ENT-Maxillofacial Surgery Department of IRCCS Casa Sollievo della Sofferenza in San Giovanni Rotondo. This multi-center approach was specifically designed to minimize selection and characterization bias among patients. The NPS is calculated based on polyp size, with scores ranging from 0 to 4 assigned to each nasal cavity. The total NPS reflects the severity of the condition, with higher scores indicating more severe nasal obstruction and polyp burden.

2.3. The Sino-Nasal Outcome Test (SNOT-22)

The Sino-Nasal Outcome Test (SNOT-22), developed at Washington University in St. Louis, MO, USA, was utilized to evaluate the quality of life (QoL) of patients suffering from CRSwNP. This questionnaire consists of 22 items, each rated on a scale from 0 (no symptom) to 5 (the worst possible symptom). The cumulative score can range from 0 to 110, with higher scores signifying a greater impact on quality of life due to nasal and sinus symptoms [15].

2.4. The Numeric Rating Scale (NRS)

The Numeric Rating Scale (NRS) was utilized to promptly gauge the patients' subjective perception of the disease. This metric is graded on a scale ranging from 0 ("no problem") to 10 ("worst possible perception"). Scores are classified into three categories: 0–3 = mild symptoms; 4–7 = moderate symptoms; and 8–10 = severe symptoms [16].

2.5. The Lund–Mackay CT Score

An initial assessment of the facial mass was carried out utilizing Computed Tomography (CT), with the Lund–Mackay CT score utilized for evaluation. This scoring system evaluates the opacity of each paranasal sinus, assigning a score between 0 (indicating no opacity) and 2 (indicating complete opacity). The total Lund–Mackay score ranges from 0 to 24, with higher scores indicative of a more significant sino-nasal disease burden. The cumulative score spans from 0 to 24, with higher scores indicating more pronounced opacity [17].

2.6. The Visual Analog Scale (VAS): Assessment of Sense of Smell

Sense of smell in the patients with chronic rhinosinusitis with nasal polyps (CRSwNP) was evaluated using the Visual Analog Scale (VAS) for olfactory function.

The VAS is a widely used, validated tool that allows patients to subjectively rate their ability to smell on a scale of 0 to 100, with 0 indicating complete anosmia (no sense of smell) and 100 indicating normal olfactory function.

This scale can take various formats, but the most common version consists of a 10 cm horizontal line with "no pain" labeled at one end and "worst pain ever" at the other. Patients indicate the intensity of their pain by placing a mark on the VAS line. The severity of the pain is directly proportional to the distance, in centimeters, from the "no pain" end of the VAS line to the patient's mark [18].

2.7. Safety Assessments

Adverse events were monitored throughout this study's duration. Safety assessments included tracking injection site reactions, allergic responses, and any unexpected health issues. The participants were instructed to report any adverse effects immediately, and serious adverse events were reported to the institutional review boards in accordance with the regulatory requirements.

2.8. Ethical Considerations

This study was conducted in adherence with the Good Clinical Practice guidelines. Ethical approval was obtained from the relevant ethics committees before the initiation of this study, and informed consent was secured from all of the participants.

3. Results

3.1. Clinical Sample, Enrollment Criteria, and Treatment with Dupilumab

The clinical cohort consisted of 40 patients, of whom 38 had completed treatment for a minimum of 6 months. However, one patient discontinued treatment after the second drug administration due to psycho-emotional issues, and another was excluded due to hypereosinophilia, necessitating a switch to mepolizumab. The clinical outcomes were evaluated in this sample, comprising 31 males and 9 females aged between 31 and

79 years old, all diagnosed with chronic rhinosinusitis with nasal polyposis. A total of 45% percent of the patients had a clinical diagnosis of asthma, with 21% classified as moderate and 79% as mild. Forty percent of patients suffered from inhalant allergies, while seven had NSAID-ERD (nonsteroidal-anti-inflammatory-drug-exacerbated respiratory disease). Patients received treatment with Dupixent (dupilumab), with a 300 mg solution for subcutaneous injection administered every 2 weeks. Each single-use pre-filled pen contained 300 mg of dupilumab in 2 mL of solution (150 mg/mL). This treatment was complemented by intranasal topical corticosteroid therapy using mometasone furoate nasal spray, administered twice daily for a total of 200 mg/day. To be eligible for this study, patients had to be at least 18 years old, diagnosed with chronic rhinosinusitis with severe nasal polyposis, and have a total score on the endoscopic nasal polyposis score (NPS) ≥ 5, along with a SNOT-22 score ≥ 50. Previous treatments had to have failed due to lack of efficacy, discontinuation of systemic corticosteroid therapy, and/or a lack of response or relapse following surgery. Seventy-eight percent of the patients examined had undergone at least one Functional Endoscopic Sinus Surgery (FESS). The patient assessment included the Nasal Polyp Score (NPS), the Lund–Mackay CT score, peripheral eosinophilia, total IgE, and the impact on quality of life (QoL) assessed through the Sino-Nasal Outcome Test questionnaire (SNOT-22) from Washington University in St. Louis, MO, USA. The overall impact of the disease was evaluated using the Numerical Rating Scale (NRS). The standard guidelines on the patient recruitment flow and the different types of biases are presented in the following flow chart (Figure 1).

3.2. Examining the Distribution of CRSwNP Based on Age and Gender

Our study enrolled 40 patients diagnosed with CRSwNP to analyze the clinical efficacy of dupilumab. The sample comprised 45% female and 55% male patients (Table 1). The mean age of the enrolled patients was 57.4 years for men and 56.7 years for women (Table 1). The median age of the entire group of patients analyzed was 57.1. The demographic data for the CRSwNP patients enrolled in this study are detailed in Table 1. Among the enrolled CRSwNP patients, 40% were asthmatic (Table 1), with 21% experiencing moderate asthma and 79% experiencing mild asthma. Additionally, seven patients had NSAID-ERD (nonsteroidal-anti-inflammatory-drug-exacerbated respiratory disease), and 40% of patients experienced inhalant allergies (Table 1).

Table 1. Baseline demographic and clinical characteristics of patients with CRSwNP.

Characteristic	Total Cohort (*n* = 40)
Age, mean (SD)	57.1 (14.3)
Gender, n (%)	
Male	22 (55%)
Female	18 (45%)
Race/ethnicity, n (%)	
Caucasian	34 (85%)
Hispanic	3 (7.5%)
Black	2 (5%)
Other	1 (2.5%)
Comorbidities, n (%)	
Asthma	16 (40%)
NSAID-exacerbated respiratory disease (NSAID-ERD)	7 (17.5%)
Inhalant allergies	16 (40%)
Baseline clinical scores, mean (SD)	
Nasal Polyp Score (NPS)	6.9 (1.0)
Sino-Nasal Outcome Test (SNOT-22)	53.6 (22.4)
Numeric Rating Scale (NRS)	7.7 (1.2)
Visual Analog Scale (VAS) for smell	72.3 (22.0)

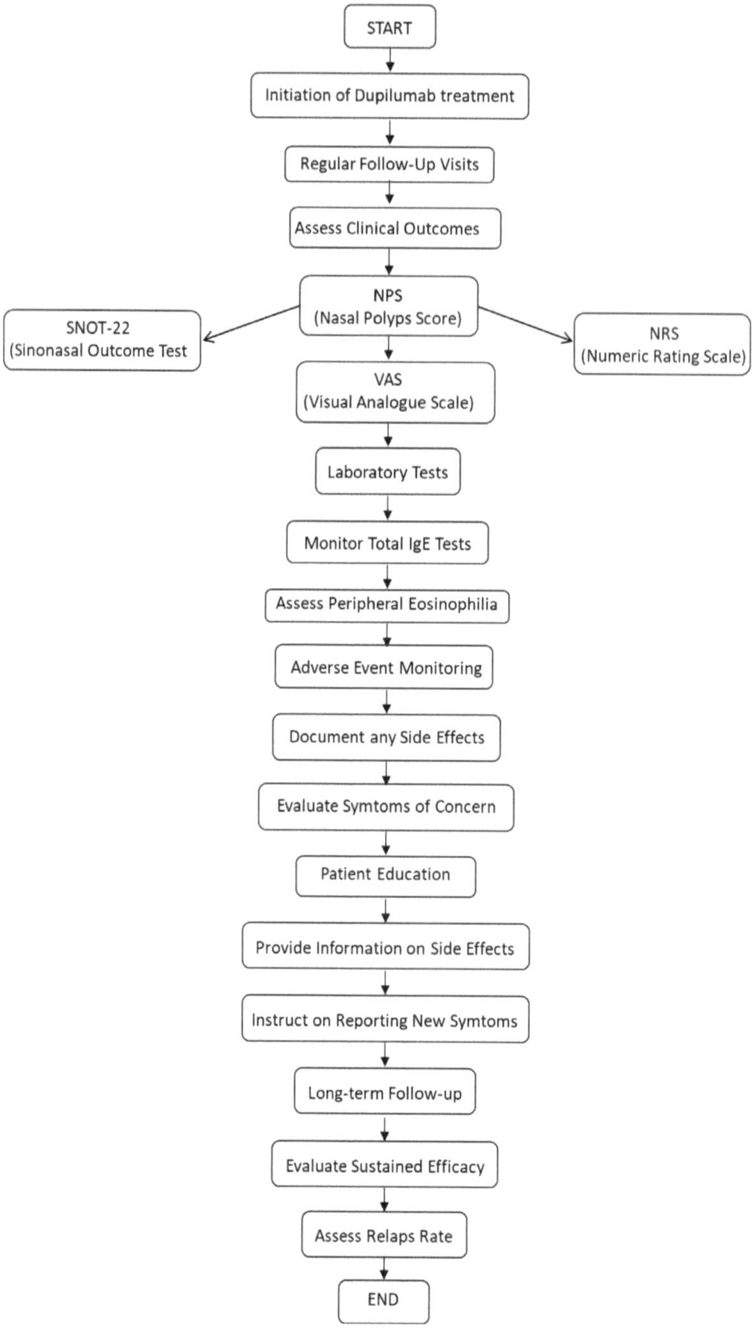

Figure 1. Flow chart summarizing the follow-up process for patients receiving dupilumab treatment. It outlines the key steps, including the initiation of treatment, assessments during regular follow-up visits, and the monitoring of clinical outcomes, laboratory tests, and patient education.

3.3. Dupilumab Treatment Led to Improvements in SNOT-22, NPS, NRS, and VAS Parameters in Patients with CRSwNP

The patients underwent a 42-week treatment course with dupilumab, during which their SNOT-22, NPS, NRS, and VAS parameters were evaluated, with their total IgE levels assessed at 16-week intervals. The initial parameter assessed was the score in the Sino-Nasal Outcome Test 22 (SNOT-22), a measure impacting surgical outcomes in chronic rhinosinusitis (CRS). Following 42 weeks of dupilumab treatment, their SNOT-22 values decreased by approximately 4.5 times. Specifically, the mean SNOT-22 score at baseline was 53.64 ± 22.39, which reduced to 11.85 ± 8.73 after 42 weeks (Figure 2A). Subsequent evaluation involved the Nasal Polyp Score (NPS) determined via nasal endoscopy, reflecting the extent of nasal polyp involvement. This parameter significantly improved after 42 weeks of dupilumab treatment, with the mean NPS decreasing from approximately 6.9 ± 1 at baseline to 2.8 ± 1 after 42 weeks, an approximately 2.4-fold reduction (Figure 2B). The patients' perceived symptom severity, as measured by the Numeric Rating Scale (NRS), also improved by approximately threefold after 42 weeks of dupilumab treatment, with their scores decreasing from 7.73 ± 1.2 at baseline to 2.5 ± 1 at 42 weeks (Figure 2C). Finally, the Visual Analog Scale (VAS), used to assess pain intensity, showed significant improvement after 42 weeks of dupilumab treatment, with the baseline scores averaging 72.3 ± 22 and reducing to 36.75 ± 14 after 42 weeks (Figure 2D).

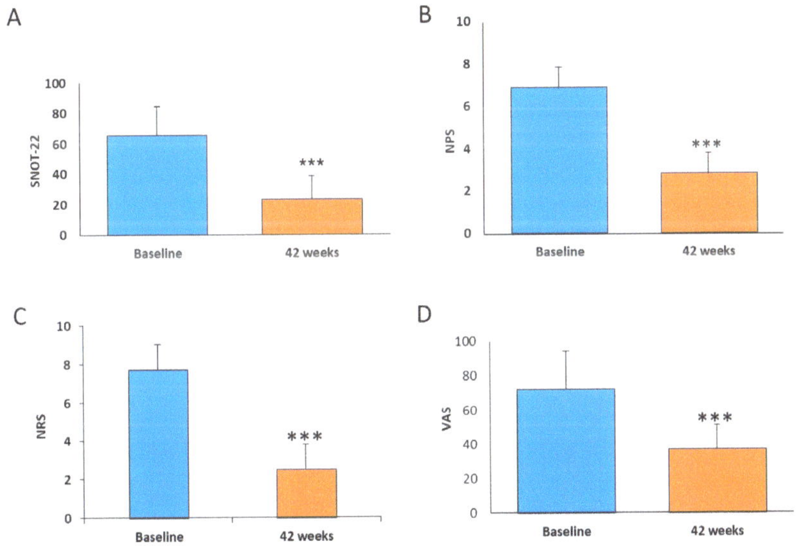

Figure 2. These figures depict the average values in (**A**) SNOT-22, (**B**) NPS, (**C**) NRS, and (**D**) VAS measured in 40 patients with CRSwNP undergoing dupilumab treatment for 42 weeks. These values were compared to the baseline averages. Data are shown as means ± SD from 40 patients (*** $p < 0.0001$).

3.4. Assessment of Total IgE Levels in CRSwNP Patients Treated with Dupilumab for 42 Weeks

Total IgE levels were evaluated after 42 weeks of treatment with dupilumab. Notably, there was a significant increase of approximately 2.1 times in the patients undergoing treatment compared to baseline. Specifically, the total blood IgE data decreased from a baseline value of 150.74 kU/L to 70.15 kU/L at 24 weeks ($p < 0.0001$), as shown in Figure 3.

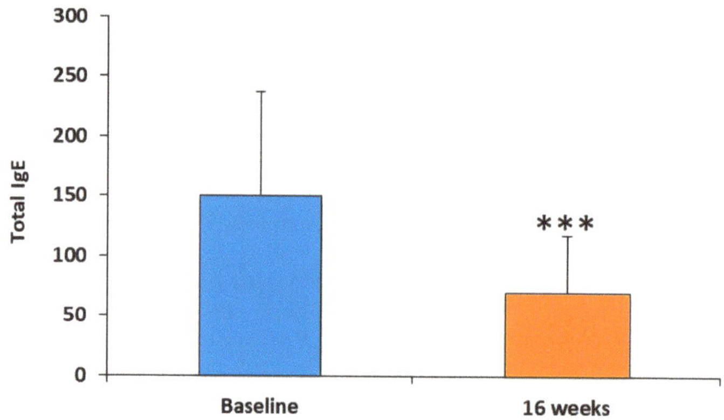

Figure 3. The histogram illustrates the mean values of total IgE assessed in 40 patients with CRSwNP treated with 300 m of dupilumab g for 24 weeks. The data were compared to the baseline mean values and are presented as means ± SD from 40 patients (*** $p < 0.0001$).

3.5. *Assessment of Peripheral Eosinophilia in CRSwNP Patients Treated with Dupilumab for 16 Weeks*

Peripheral eosinophilia levels were examined after 16 weeks of treatment. Notably, there was a significant increase of approximately 1.3 times in the patients undergoing treatment compared to baseline. The mean value of peripheral eosinophils was 0.24 ± 0.21 cells/µL at baseline and 0.32 ± 0.21 cells/µL at 16 weeks (Figure 4).

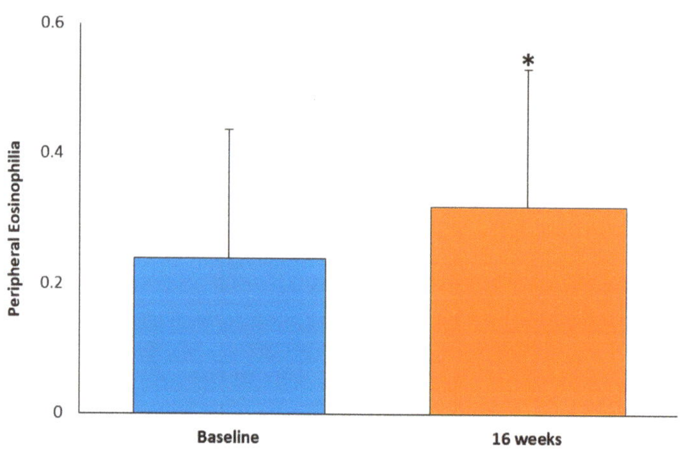

Figure 4. The data were compared to the baseline mean values and are presented as means SD from 40 patients (* $p < 0.05$).

3.6. *Statistical Analysis*

A statistical analysis was performed using Microsoft Excel (San Diego, CA, USA), and Matplotlib. All of the data are presented as means ± SD (standard deviation). The normality of the data distribution was assessed using the Anderson–Darling and Kolmogorov–Smirnov tests. Student's *t*-test and the Mann–Whitney U test were utilized to compare variables as appropriate. A *p*-value < 0.05 was considered statistically significant. The average age of the patients was 56.72 ± 12.68 years old. At the outset of the treatment, the patients had a mean Lund–Mackay CT Score of 23.64 ± 1.32. Please note that verification of this information is pending as we await additional data.

4. Discussion

Our study demonstrated that dupilumab, a monoclonal antibody targeting IL-4 and IL-13 signaling, was highly effective in improving the clinical outcomes of patients with chronic rhinosinusitis with nasal polyps (CRSwNP). Specifically, significant improvements were observed in all of the parameters assessed, including the Sino-Nasal Outcome Test (SNOT-22), the Nasal Polyp Score (NPS), the Numeric Rating Scale (NRS), the Visual Analog Scale (VAS), total IgE levels, and peripheral eosinophilia after 42 weeks of treatment.

These findings indicate that dupilumab effectively addresses the underlying type 2 inflammatory pathways characteristic of CRSwNP. Type 2 inflammation, driven by cytokines such as IL-4, IL-5, and IL-13, is a hallmark of CRSwNP. These cytokines promote eosinophil recruitment and activation, leading to tissue damage, mucus hypersecretion, and nasal polyp formation. Through blocking IL-13 signaling, dupilumab disrupts this cycle of inflammation, reducing nasal polyps and improving mucosal function [19–21].

Studies have demonstrated that while dupilumab effectively reduces the symptoms of conditions associated with type 2 inflammation, such as asthma and chronic rhinosinusitis with nasal polyps (CRSwNP), its impact on IgE levels is more nuanced. Specifically, dupilumab has been shown to lead to a reduction in IgE levels in some patients, but this effect is not universal. It is essential to clarify that the clinical benefits observed in our study were not solely dependent on changes in IgE levels; rather, they reflect a more comprehensive modulation of the immune response. Research indicates that while dupilumab can inhibit IgE production by blocking IL-4 and IL-13 signaling, it does not eliminate IgE from the circulation entirely.

For instance, in a study by Hoshino et al., the authors noted that although dupilumab treatment resulted in significant clinical improvements, the overall total IgE levels varied among patients, with some experiencing no significant change in their IgE levels despite symptom relief [22]. Similarly, Castro et al. (2018) found that dupilumab reduced exacerbations and improved asthma control in patients, but their total IgE levels did not correlate directly with the clinical outcomes [23]. These findings suggest that the clinical benefits of dupilumab are not solely dependent on changes in total IgE levels.

By addressing the underlying type 2 inflammatory pathways rather than directly lowering IgE levels, dupilumab offers a unique therapeutic strategy for managing conditions characterized by eosinophilic inflammation and IgE-mediated responses.

The observed reduction in the total IgE levels in our study is consistent with dupilumab's effect on B cells, inhibiting the switch to IgE production. IL-4 and IL-13 are critical cytokines for inducing IgE class switching, and dupilumab's ability to reduce IgE levels in patients with CRSwNP has been noted in prior studies. These findings elucidate how the modulation of IgE may correlate with the overall reduction in allergic symptoms, particularly in patients with concomitant allergies, further supporting the therapeutic role of dupilumab in addressing type 2 inflammation beyond asthma and atopic dermatitis [24–28].

Our study showed a transient increase in peripheral eosinophilia after 16 weeks of treatment, a phenomenon also observed in previous clinical trials. While the increase in eosinophil counts may initially raise concern, it is important to note that dupilumab's mechanism involves inhibiting eosinophil migration into the tissue rather than directly reducing blood eosinophil counts. We acknowledge that this transient increase may be a counterintuitive aspect of dupilumab's efficacy and that it merits further exploration in future studies. This explains the observed peripheral eosinophilia, as circulating eosinophils are no longer being recruited into the inflamed nasal tissues. Previous studies have demonstrated that despite transient changes, eosinophil outcomes continue to improve, and eosinophil levels eventually return to baseline. Furthermore, eosinophilia-related adverse events were rare and did not compromise the treatment, a finding consistent with the literature [29].

Our results align with those from the pivotal SINUS-24 trials, where dupilumab significantly reduced polyp size, improved symptoms, and enhanced patients' quality of life. However, our study showed a slightly greater reduction in the NPS compared to these trials [30]. One possible explanation may be differences in the baseline characteristics of the patient population, as our cohort included a higher percentage of patients with comorbid asthma, a condition strongly associated with more severe type 2 inflammation. This highlights the need for a stratified approach in future studies to understand the varying impacts of dupilumab among different patient subgroups better. The pronounced effect of dupilumab in patients with both CRSwNP and asthma has been highlighted in previous studies, improving not only nasal symptoms but also respiratory function. The marked improvement in quality of life, as indicated by reductions in SNOT-22 and VAS scores, is a critical outcome for CRSwNP patients. These improvements are particularly significant given the high disease burden associated with CRSwNP, which often leads to impaired sleep, loss of smell, and reduced daily functioning [31–33].

Dupilumab's ability to restore olfactory function, as seen in our study and corroborated by others, addresses one of its most challenging symptoms [25,34,35].

As dupilumab continues to demonstrate efficacy in reducing nasal polyps and improving patient outcomes, the treatment landscape for CRSwNP is becoming more defined. However, several challenges remain. Relapse of CRS after discontinuing biologic therapy is a critical issue [36].

Biologics primarily target inflammatory pathways to reduce symptoms and prevent polyp recurrence, but they do not cure the underlying disease [37]. Therefore, the discontinuation of treatment may lead to the reactivation of inflammatory processes and a recurrence of symptoms, as seen in some patients after biologic withdrawal [38,39].

Another key consideration is the economic impact of biologic therapies. Dupilumab's high cost may limit its accessibility, especially in healthcare systems with constrained budgets. To enhance the clinical applicability of dupilumab, identifying biomarkers that can predict which patients will benefit most from dupilumab could optimize its use and make it more cost-effective [40–44].

Future research should focus on defining the patient selection criteria, possibly through the development of predictive biomarkers for the treatment response. Additionally, a more detailed methodology in future studies will be critical for establishing the reproducibility and robustness of our findings. Long-term studies should assess the sustained efficacy and safety of dupilumab, particularly regarding eosinophilia and other potential immune-related effects.

5. Conclusions

Our study provides preliminary evidence that dupilumab may offer therapeutic benefits in patients with CRSwNP, showing significant improvements in symptom severity, nasal polyp size, and quality of life measures. While these findings suggest the potential effectiveness of dupilumab in targeting type 2 inflammation in CRSwNP, this study's observational design and absence of a control group limit the ability to draw definitive conclusions about causal efficacy. Further randomized controlled trials with larger, more diverse populations and extended follow-up periods are necessary to confirm these findings and establish dupilumab as a standard treatment option in CRSwNP management.

Study Limitations

Several limitations should be considered when interpreting the findings of this study. First, the sample size was relatively small, with only 40 patients included, which may limit the generalizability of the results to larger and more diverse populations. Additionally, this was a single-center study, and the patient demographics may not reflect those of broader populations, potentially limiting the external validity of our findings.

Second, while we monitored key clinical parameters such as symptom scores, polyp size, and biomarkers (e.g., total IgE, peripheral eosinophilia), other important markers of inflammation and disease progression, such as specific tissue biopsy analyses, were not incorporated. A more comprehensive understanding of the molecular and histopathological changes associated with treatment would have provided deeper insight into the mechanisms behind the clinical improvements observed.

Third, this study's follow-up period was limited. While we were able to capture the short-term outcomes, a longer follow-up would be necessary to assess the sustained efficacy of dupilumab over time, as well as the potential for disease recurrence after the discontinuation of treatment.

Finally, the absence of a control group in this cohort limits our ability to directly compare the outcomes of patients receiving dupilumab with those receiving other standard treatments such as corticosteroids or surgical interventions. Future studies should include randomized controlled trials to assess the comparative effectiveness of biologic treatments in CRS more rigorously.

Author Contributions: Conceptualization, N.L. (Nicola Lombardo), G.L.P. and N.L. (Nadia Lobello); methodology, C.P.; software, A.R.; validation, N.L. (Nicola Lombardo), D.R., C.P. and A.R.; formal analysis, N.L. (Nadia Lobello) and N.L. (Nicola Lombardo); investigation, E.C.; resources, G.L.P.; data curation, N.L. (Nadia Lobello); writing—original draft preparation, E.C.; writing—review and editing, E.C.; visualization, A.D. and N.L. (Nicola Lombardo); supervision, N.L. (Nicola Lombardo); project administration, A.R.; funding acquisition, D.R. All authors have read and agreed to the published version of the manuscript.

Funding: This research received no external funding.

Institutional Review Board Statement: This study was conducted in accordance with the Declaration of Helsinki and approved by the local Ethical Committee of Calabria Region (Catanzaro, Italy; document 182—20 May 2021).

Informed Consent Statement: Informed consent was obtained from all of the subjects involved in this study.

Data Availability Statement: Data are contained within the article.

Conflicts of Interest: The authors declare no conflicts of interest.

References

1. Zucoloto, N.N.; de Aguiar, F.S.; Lopes, N.M.D.; Garcia, E.C.D.; Romano, F.R.; Bezerra, T.F.P.; Lima, W.T.A.; Fornazieri, M.A. Exploring the impact of inflammatory endotypes on olfactory function and quality of life in chronic rhinosinusitis patients. *Braz. J. Otorhinolaryngol.* **2023**, *90*, 101364. [CrossRef] [PubMed] [PubMed Central]
2. Cho, S.H.; Hamilos, D.L.; Han, D.H.; Laidlaw, T.M. Phenotypes of Chronic Rhinosinusitis. *J. Allergy Clin. Immunol. Pract.* **2020**, *8*, 1505–1511. [CrossRef] [PubMed]
3. Ostovar, A.; Fokkens, W.J.; Vahdat, K.; Raeisi, A.; Mallahzadeh, A.; Farrokhi, S. Epidemiology of chronic rhinosinusitis in Bushehr, southwestern region of Iran: A GA2LEN study. *Rhinology* **2019**, *57*, 43–48. [CrossRef] [PubMed]
4. Schwitzguébel, A.J.; Jandus, P.; Lacroix, J.S.; Seebach, J.D.; Harr, T. Immunoglobulin deficiency in patients with chronic rhinosinusitis: Systematic review of the literature and meta-analysis. *J. Allergy Clin. Immunol.* **2015**, *136*, 1523–1531. [CrossRef] [PubMed]
5. Boita, M.; Bucca, C.; Riva, G.; Heffler, E.; Rolla, G. Release of Type 2 Cytokines by Epithelial Cells of Nasal Polyps. *J. Immunol. Res.* **2016**, *2016*, 2643297. [CrossRef]
6. Chiarella, E.; Lombardo, N.; Lobello, N.; Piazzetta, G.L.; Morrone, H.L.; Mesuraca, M.; Bond, H.M. Deficit in Adipose Differentiation in Mesenchymal Stem Cells Derived from Chronic Rhinosinusitis Nasal Polyps Compared to Nasal Mucosal Tissue. *Int. J. Mol. Sci.* **2020**, *21*, 9214. [CrossRef]
7. Mesuraca, M.; Nisticò, C.; Lombardo, N.; Piazzetta, G.L.; Lobello, N.; Chiarella, E. Cellular and Biochemical Characterization of Mesenchymal Stem Cells from Killian Nasal Polyp. *Int. J. Mol. Sci.* **2022**, *23*, 13214. [CrossRef]
8. Won, H.K.; Kim, Y.C.; Kang, M.G.; Park, H.K.; Lee, S.E.; Kim, M.H.; Yang, M.S.; Chang, Y.S.; Cho, S.H.; Song, W.J. Age-related prevalence of chronic rhinosinusitis and nasal polyps and their relationships with asthma onset. *Ann. Allergy Asthma Immunol.* **2018**, *120*, 389–394. [CrossRef]
9. Seybt, M.W.; McMains, K.C.; Kountakis, S.E. The prevalence and effect of asthma on adults with chronic rhinosinusitis. *Ear Nose Throat J.* **2007**, *86*, 409–411. [CrossRef]
10. Wilson, K.F.; McMains, K.C.; Orlandi, R.R. The association between allergy and chronic rhinosinusitis with and without nasal polyps: An evidence-based review with recommendations. *Int. Forum Allergy Rhinol.* **2014**, *4*, 93–103. [CrossRef]
11. Lombardo, N.; Piazzetta, G.L.; Lobello, N.; Cicala, G.; Patafi, M.; Benincasa, A.T.; Pelaia, C.; Chiarella, E.; Pelaia, G. Real-Life Effects of Omalizumab on Chronic Rhinosinusitis with Nasal Polyposis. *J. Pers. Med.* **2023**, *14*, 3. [CrossRef] [PubMed]

12. Bachert, C.; Sousa, A.R.; Lund, V.J.; Scadding, G.K.; Gevaert, P.; Nasser, S.; Durham, S.R.; Cornet, M.E.; Kariyawasam, H.H.; Gilbert, J.; et al. Reduced need for surgery in severe nasal polyposis with mepolizumab: Randomized trial. *J. Allergy Clin. Immunol.* **2017**, *140*, 1024–1031.e14. [CrossRef] [PubMed]
13. Pelaia, G.; Vatrella, A.; Busceti, M.T.; Gallelli, L.; Preianò, M.; Lombardo, N.; Terracciano, R.; Maselli, R. Role of biologics in severe eosinophilic asthma—Focus on reslizumab. *Ther. Clin. Risk Manag.* **2016**, *12*, 1075–1082. [CrossRef] [PubMed]
14. Piazzetta, G.L.; Lobello, N.; Chiarella, E.; Rizzuti, A.; Pelaia, C.; Pelaia, G.; Lombardo, N. Targeting IL-4 and IL-13 Receptors on Eosinophils in CRSwNP Patients: The Clinical Efficacy of Dupilumab. *J. Pers. Med.* **2023**, *13*, 1404. [CrossRef]
15. Gallo, S.; Russo, F.; Mozzanica, F.; Preti, A.; Bandi, F.; Costantino, C.; Gera, R.; Ottaviani, F.; Castelnuovo, P. Prognostic value of the Sinonasal Outcome Test 22 (SNOT-22) in chronic rhinosinusitis. *Acta Otorhinolaryngol. Ital.* **2020**, *40*, 113–121. [CrossRef]
16. Hjermstad, M.J.; Fayers, P.M.; Haugen, D.F.; Caraceni, A.; Hanks, G.W.; Loge, J.H.; Fainsinger, R.; Aass, N.; Kaasa, S.; European Palliative Care Research Collaborative (EPCRC). Studies comparing Numerical Rating Scales, Verbal Rating Scales, and Visual Analogue Scales for assessment of pain intensity in adults: A systematic literature review. *J. Pain Symptom Manag.* **2011**, *41*, 1073–1093. [CrossRef]
17. Hopkins, C.; Browne, J.P.; Slack, R.; Lund, V.; Brown, P. The Lund-Mackay staging system for chronic rhinosinusitis: How is it used and what does it predict? *Otolaryngol. Head Neck Surg.* **2007**, *137*, 555–561. [CrossRef]
18. Alobid, I.; Calvo-Henríquez, C.; Viveros-Díez, P.; López-Chacón, M.; Rojas-Lechuga, M.J.; Langdon, C.; Marin, C.; Mullol, J. Validation of Visual Analogue Scale for loss of smell as a quick test in chronic rhinosinusitis with nasal polyps. *J. Investig. Allergol. Clin. Immunol.* **2023**, *advance online publication*. [CrossRef]
19. Hoy, S.M. Dupilumab: A Review in Chronic Rhinosinusitis with Nasal Polyps. *Drugs* **2020**, *80*, 711–717. [CrossRef]
20. Boscke, R.; Heidemann, M.; Bruchhage, K.L. Dupilumab for chronic rhinosinusitis with nasal polyps: Real-life retrospective 12-month effectiveness data. *Rhinology* **2023**, *61*, 203–213. [CrossRef]
21. Peters, A.T.; Wagenmann, M.; Bernstein, J.A.; Khan, A.H.; Nash, S.; Jacob-Nara, J.A.; Siddiqui, S.; Rowe, P.J.; Deniz, Y. Dupilumab efficacy in patients with chronic rhinosinusitis with nasal polyps with and without allergic rhinitis. *Allergy Asthma Proc.* **2023**, *44*, 265–274. [CrossRef] [PubMed]
22. Hoshino, M.; Akitsu, K.; Kubota, K.; Ohtawa, J. Efficacy of a house dust mite sublingual immunotherapy tablet as add-on dupilumab in asthma with rhinitis. *Allergol. Int.* **2022**, *71*, 490–497. [CrossRef] [PubMed]
23. Castro, M.; Corren, J.; Pavord, I.D.; Maspero, J.; Wenzel, S.; Rabe, K.F.; Busse, W.W.; Ford, L.; Sher, L.; FitzGerald, J.M.; et al. Dupilumab Efficacy and Safety in Moderate-to-Severe Uncontrolled Asthma. *N. Engl. J. Med.* **2018**, *378*, 2486–2496. [CrossRef] [PubMed]
24. Jansen, F.; Becker, B.; Eden, J.K.; Breda, P.C.; Hot, A.; Oqueka, T.; Betz, C.S.; Hoffmann, A.S. Dupilumab (Dupixent.) tends to be an effective therapy for uncontrolled severe chronic rhinosinusitis with nasal polyps: Real data of a single-centered, retrospective single-arm longitudinal study from a university hospital in Germany. *Eur. Arch. Otorhinolaryngol.* **2023**, *280*, 1741–1755. [CrossRef] [PubMed]
25. Mullol, J.; Bachert, C.; Amin, N.; Desrosiers, M.; Hellings, P.W.; Han, J.K.; Jankowski, R.; Vodicka, J.; Gevaert, P.; Daizadeh, N.; et al. Olfactory Outcomes with Dupilumab in Chronic Rhinosinusitis with Nasal Polyps. *J. Allergy Clin. Immunol. Pract.* **2022**, *10*, 1086–1095.e5. [CrossRef]
26. Ottaviano, G.; Saccardo, T.; Roccuzzo, G.; Bernardi, R.; Chicco, A.D.; Pendolino, A.L.; Scarpa, B.; Mairani, E.; Nicolai, P. Effectiveness of Dupilumab in the Treatment of Patients with Uncontrolled Severe CRSwNP: A "Real-Life" Observational Study in Na.ve and Post-Surgical Patients. *J. Pers. Med.* **2022**, *12*, 1526. [CrossRef]
27. De Corso, E.; Pasquini, E.; Trimarchi, M.; La Mantia, I.; Pagella, F.; Ottaviano, G.; Garzaro, M.; Pipolo, C.; Torretta, S.; Seccia, V.; et al. Dupilumab in the treatment of severe uncontrolled chronic rhinosinusitis with nasal polyps (CRSwNP): A multicentric observational Phase IV real-life study (DUPIREAL). *Allergy* **2023**, *online ahead of print*. [CrossRef]
28. Wang, Y.; Jorizzo, J.L. Retrospective analysis of adverse events with dupilumab reported to the United States Food and Drug Administration. *J. Am. Acad. Dermatol.* **2021**, *84*, 1010–1014. [CrossRef]
29. Li, S.H.; Nehme, K.F.; Moshkovich, A.; Suh, L.; Pawlowski, A.; Ali, Y.; Patel, G.B.; Kuang, F.L.; Peters, A.T. Eosinophilia and Adverse Effects of Dupilumab for Respiratory Indications: A Real-World Setting. *J. Allergy Clin. Immunol. Pract.* **2024**. [CrossRef]
30. Bachert, C.; Han, J.K.; Desrosiers, M.; Hellings, P.W.; Amin, N.; Lee, S.E.; Mullol, J.; Greos, L.S.; Bosso, J.V.; Laidlaw, T.M.; et al. Efficacy and safety of dupilumab in patients with severe chronic rhinosinusitis with nasal polyps (LIBERTY NP SINUS-24 and LIBERTY NP SINUS-52): Results from two multicentre, randomised, double-blind, placebo-controlled, parallel-group phase 3 trials. *Lancet* **2019**, *394*, 1638–1650. [CrossRef]
31. Maspero, J.F.; Khan, A.H.; Philpott, C.; Hellings, P.W.; Hopkins, C.; Wagenmann, M.; Siddiqui, S.; Msihid, J.; Nash, S.; Chuang, C.C.; et al. Health-Related Quality of Life Impairment Among Patients with Severe Chronic Rhinosinusitis with Nasal Polyps in the SINUS-24 Trial. *J. Asthma Allergy* **2023**, *16*, 323–332. [CrossRef] [PubMed]
32. Ferri, S.; Montagna, C.; Casini, M.; Malvezzi, L.; Pirola, F.; Russo, E.; Racca, F.; Messina, M.R.; Puggioni, F.; Nappi, E.; et al. Sleep quality burden in chronic rhinosinusitis with nasal polyps and its modulation by dupilumab. *Ann. Allergy Asthma Immunol.* **2024**, *132*, 69–75. [CrossRef] [PubMed]
33. Macchi, A.; Giorli, A.; Cantone, E.; Carlotta Pipolo, G.; Arnone, F.; Barbone, U.; Bertazzoni, G.; Bianchini, C.; Ciofalo, A.; Cipolla, F.; et al. Sense of smell in chronic rhinosinusitis: A multicentric study on 811 patients. *Front. Allergy* **2023**, *4*, 1083964. [CrossRef] [PubMed]

34. La Mantia, I.; Grigaliute, E.; Ragusa, M.; Cocuzza, S.; Radulesco, T.; Saibene, A.M.; Calvo-Henriquez, C.; Fakhry, N.; Michel, J.; Maniaci, A. Effectiveness and rapidity on olfatory fuction recovery in CRS patients treated with Dupilumab: A real life prospective controlled study. *Eur. Arch. Otorhinolaryngol.* **2024**, *281*, 219–226. [CrossRef] [PubMed]
35. Cantone, E.; De Corso, E.; Ricciardiello, F.; Di Nola, C.; Grimaldi, G.; Allocca, V.; Motta, G. Olfaction Recovery following Dupilumab Is Independent of Nasal Polyp Reduction in CRSwNP. *J. Pers. Med.* **2022**, *12*, 1215. [CrossRef]
36. Kim, D.H.; Kim, S.W. Considerations for the Use of Biologic Agents in Patients with Chronic Rhinosinusitis with Nasal Polyposis. *Clin. Exp. Otorhinolaryngol.* **2021**, *14*, 245–246; Erratum in *Clin. Exp. Otorhinolaryngol.* **2021**, *14*, 435. [CrossRef]
37. Bellocchi, G.; Loperfido, A.; Passali, F.M.; Millarelli, S.; Velletrani, G.; Perla, M.; Di Michele, L.; Di Girolamo, S. Biologics in severe uncontrolled chronic rhinosinusitis with nasal polyps: A bicentric experience. *Acta Biomed.* **2023**, *94*, e2023227.
38. Sima, Y.; Zhang, J.; Zheng, M.; Zhao, Y.; Wang, X.; Zhang, L. Revision surgery versus biologic treatment with omalizumab in recurrent chronic rhinosinusitis with nasal polyps: An analysis of cost-utility and clinical outcomes. *World Allergy Organ. J.* **2023**, *16*, 100846. [CrossRef]
39. Chiarella, E.; Lombardo, N.; Lobello, N.; Aloisio, A.; Aragona, T.; Pelaia, C.; Scicchitano, S.; Bond, H.M.; Mesuraca, M. Nasal Polyposis: Insights in Epithelial-Mesenchymal Transition and Differentiation of Polyp Mesenchymal Stem Cells. *Int. J. Mol. Sci.* **2020**, *21*, 6878. [CrossRef]
40. Brown, W.C.; Senior, B. A Critical Look at the Efficacy and Costs of Biologic Therapy for Chronic Rhinosinusitis with Nasal Polyposis. *Curr. Allergy Asthma Rep.* **2020**, *20*, 16. [CrossRef]
41. Yong, M.; Kirubalingam, K.; Desrosiers, M.Y.; Kilty, S.J.; Thamboo, A. Cost-effectiveness analysis of biologics for the treatment of chronic rhinosinusitis with nasal polyps in Canada. *Allergy Asthma Clin. Immunol.* **2023**, *19*, 90. [CrossRef] [PubMed]
42. Codispoti, C.D.; Mahdavinia, M. A call for cost-effectiveness analysis for biologic therapies in chronic rhinosinusitis with nasal polyps. *Ann. Allergy Asthma Immunol.* **2019**, *123*, 232–239. [CrossRef] [PubMed]
43. Frankenberger, H.; Wiebringhaus, R.; Paul, B.; Huber, P.; Haubner, F.; Gröger, M.; Stihl, C. The use of biologics in patients suffering from chronic rhinosinusitis with nasal polyps—A 4-year real life observation. *Eur. Arch. Otorhinolaryngol.* **2024**, *281*, 5773–5782. [CrossRef] [PubMed]
44. van der Lans, R.J.L.; Hopkins, C.; Senior, B.A.; Lund, V.J.; Reitsma, S. Biologicals and Endoscopic Sinus Surgery for Severe Uncontrolled Chronic Rhinosinusitis with Nasal Polyps: An Economic Perspective. *J. Allergy Clin. Immunol. Pract.* **2022**, *10*, 1454–1461. [CrossRef]

medicina

MDPI

Article

Development of a New Swine Model Resembling Human Empty Nose Syndrome

Dan Bi Park [1], David W. Jang [2], Do Hyun Kim [3,*,†] and Sung Won Kim [3,*,†]

[1] Postech-Catholic Biomedical Engineering Institute, College of Medicine, The Catholic University of Korea, Seoul 06591, Republic of Korea; bdb613@naver.com
[2] Department of Head and Neck Surgery & Communication Sciences, Duke University School of Medicine, Durham, NC 27710, USA; david.jang@duke.edu
[3] Department of Otolaryngology-Head and Neck Surgery, Seoul Saint Mary's Hospital, College of Medicine, The Catholic University of Korea, Seoul 06591, Republic of Korea
* Correspondence: dohyuni9292@naver.com (D.H.K.); kswent@catholic.ac.kr (S.W.K.); Tel.: +82-2-2258-6112 (D.H.K.); +82-2-2258-6216 (S.W.K.); Fax: +82-2-535-1354 (D.H.K. & S.W.K.)
† These authors contributed equally to this work.

Abstract: *Background and Objectives:* Empty nose syndrome (ENS) is a debilitating condition that often results from traumatic or iatrogenic causes, such as nasal surgery. There are various conservative and surgical treatments for ENS, but their effectiveness remains uncertain. Therefore, the development of animal models that accurately mimic human ENS is essential for advancing effective treatment strategies. *Materials and Methods:* To investigate ENS development, turbinoplasty was performed in the nasal cavity of swine, entailing partial removal of the ventral turbinate using turbinectomy scissors followed by electrocauterization. After 56 days, samples were obtained for histological and morphological analyses. *Results:* A significant reduction in the volume of the ventral turbinate in the ENS model led to an expansion of the nasal cavity. Histological analysis revealed mucosal epithelial changes similar to those observed in ENS patients, including squamous cell metaplasia, goblet cell metaplasia, submucosal fibrosis, and glandular atrophy. Biomarkers related to these histopathological features were identified, and signals potentially contributing to squamous cell metaplasia were elucidated. *Conclusions:* The swine ENS model is anticipated to be instrumental in unraveling the pathogenesis of ENS and may also be useful for evaluating the effectiveness of various treatments for ENS.

Keywords: empty nose syndrome; atrophic rhinitis; animal model; swine; turbinoplasty

1. Introduction

Empty nose syndrome (ENS) is an iatrogenic condition that develops subsequent to nasal surgery and particularly affects the turbinates. In 1994, Kern and Stenkvist coined this term to describe the marked reduction in intranasal tissue surrounding the inferior and middle turbinates [1]. ENS occurs in up to 16% of patients undergoing turbinate surgery, and patients can experience ENS months to years after the surgery [2,3].

Typically, ENS patients exhibit nasal-cavity symptoms such as excessive nasal crusting, mucosal dryness, paradoxical nasal obstruction, nosebleeds, and a mucus-filled runny nose. Less commonly, symptoms such as headache, facial pain, anosmia, difficulty breathing, disrupted sleep, and emotional disturbances including depression, anger, anxiety, fatigue, irritability, and frustration can cause serious psychological problems, even suicide [4,5]. Medical treatment for ENS is conservative, including hydrating the nasal passages with nasal saline spray or oil-based lubricants, prescribing anti-depressants, increasing fluid intake, and intermittently closing the nostrils to restore humidity [6,7]. This treatment is somewhat effective, but it is not curative. Consequently, the number of ENS patients is growing.

Recent studies have indicated that surgical interventions and mucosal regenerative strategies can lead to sustained alleviation of ENS symptoms. However, there is generally marginal clinical improvement in up to 21% of patients [8]. To develop effective ENS treatments, animal models of human ENS are needed. However, no animal model of ENS following turbinate surgery, which is the most common cause, has been reported. Therefore, in this study, we attempted to create an animal model of ENS and examined the underlying mechanisms of onset that can be targeted for the development of therapeutic strategies.

2. Materials and Methods

2.1. Ethics Approval

All animals involved in this experiment were cared for following ethical standards. All procedures were conducted in compliance with applicable ethical standards and received approval from the Institutional Animal Care and Use Committee (IACUC) of CRONEX (CRONEX-IACUC Approval No. 202309-002). They were maintained under controlled conditions in a standard laboratory setting in accordance with IACUC guidelines. Only animals that passed thorough screening for parasites and microbial infections, as per IACUC quarantine guidelines, were utilized in this study.

2.2. Surgical Procedure

The experimental procedure involved the use of a single female conventional swine weighing 40–50 kg. Because this trial was conducted as a pilot study to determine whether ENS could be induced via turbinoplasty, no sample-size calculation was performed. Turbinoplasty was performed on the left nasal cavity of the swine under isoflurane inhalational anesthesia, with the right nasal cavity serving as a control. The nasal cavity was examined using a 4 mm endoscope, and the ventral turbinate (equivalent to the human inferior turbinate) was partially removed using turbinectomy scissors. Hemostasis was achieved by cauterization of the mucosa using bayonet-type forceps and a ValleyLab Force FX™ Electrosurgical Generator (Medtronic, Minneapolis, MN, USA) at 15 W for 3–5 s. This procedure facilitated turbinate electrocauterization and bone repositioning. After 56 days, the animals were euthanized by an overdose of sodium pentobarbital injection and samples were collected to evaluate the procedure outcomes (Figure 1a). All surgical interventions were performed by a rhinology specialist.

2.3. Hematological Analysis

Blood samples were collected from the swine before turbinectomy was performed and at euthanasia and were transferred to heparin-coated tubes to separate serum and blood cells. Serum hematological parameters were analyzed using a Hitachi 7180 clinical analyzer (Hitachi clinical analyzer 7180; Hitachi, Tokyo, Japan), following the manufacturer's protocol. The obtained hematological values were compared with established normal ranges to assess abnormalities [9,10].

2.4. Scanning Electron Microscopy (SEM)

Turbinate tissue was fixed overnight using a 2.5% glutaraldehyde buffered solution and then rinsed twice with 0.1 M phosphate buffer and post-fixed with 2% osmium tetroxide for 2 h. Following fixation, the samples were dehydrated using a series of graded ethanol solutions and allowed to dry. Then, they were sputter-coated with platinum using the SMC12R-Plus system (Semian, Daejeon, Republic of Korea). Finally, the samples were examined by SEM (Regulus 8220; Hitachi).

2.5. Tissue Processing

Following euthanasia, samples were collected and fixed in 10% formalin overnight and then washed with phosphate-buffered saline (PBS). Then, the samples were decalcified in 14% ethylenediaminetetraacetic acid solution (pH 7.8) for 2 months before they were embedded in paraffin.

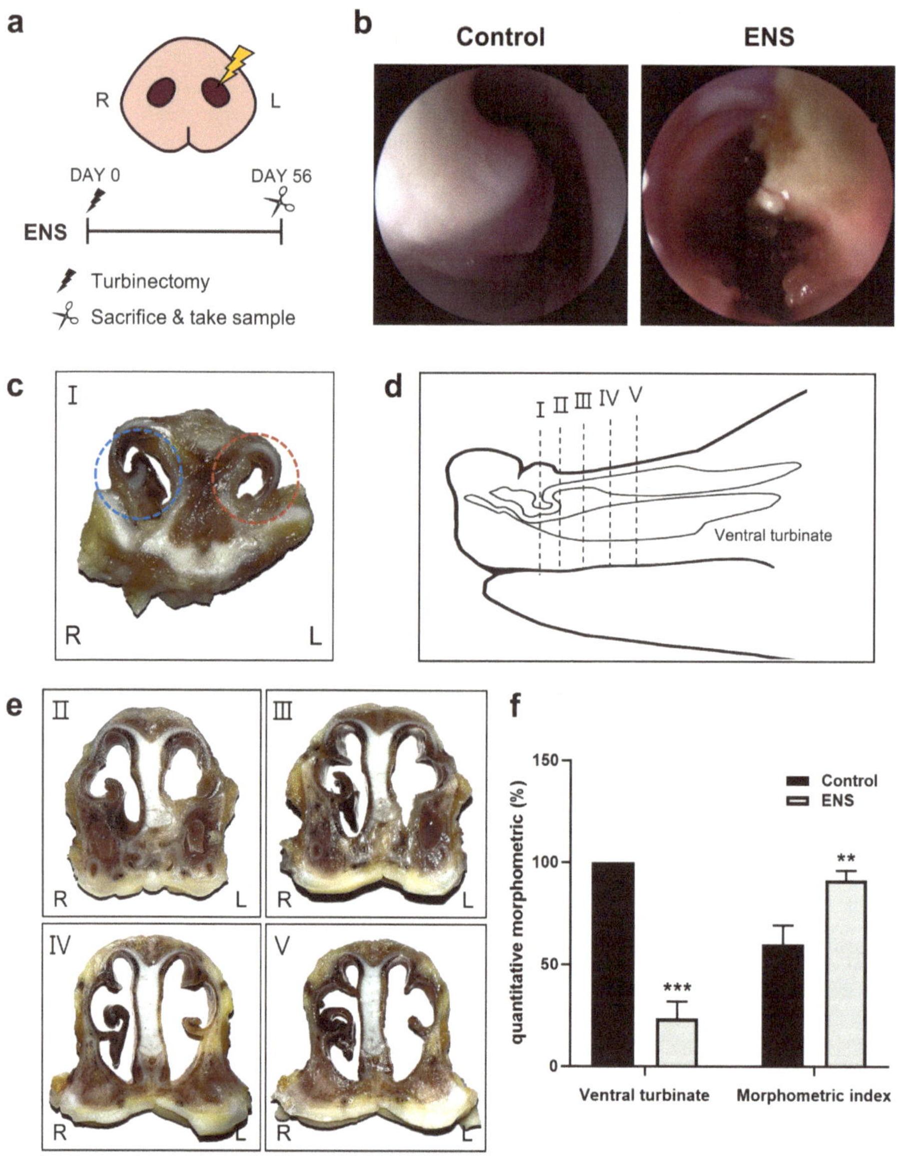

Figure 1. Morphology of the nasal cavity following turbinectomy on the swine snout. (**a**) Overview of the surgical procedure. (**b**) Endoscopic image of the swine ventral turbinate. (**c**) Cross-sectional view of the ventral turbinate: control (blue) and ENS after turbinoplasty (red). (**d**) Lateral view and cross-section of the swine snout. (**e**) Nasal cavity cross-sections at various locations. (**f**) Ventral turbinate volume and morphometric index; data are means ± standard deviation (SD) (** $p < 0.01$, *** $p < 0.001$).

2.6. Histological Analysis

The specimens were sliced into 4.0 μm thick sections, deparaffinized with xylene, and gradually rehydrated using a sequence of ethanol solutions. After deparaffinization, various sections were stained with hematoxylin and eosin (H and E; Daejung, Republic of Korea), Masson's trichrome (MT) stain kit (Abcam, Cambridge, UK), and Alcian blue (Abcam), following the manufacturers' guidelines.

2.7. Immunohistochemistry (IHC) and Immunofluorescence (IF) Analysis

Each section was subjected to heat-induced epitope retrieval in 0.01 M citrate buffer (Sigma-Aldrich, St. Louis, MO, USA), and then endogenous peroxidase activity was neutralized using 3% H_2O_2. Subsequently, the sections were blocked with 5% normal goat serum (Vector Laboratories, Newark, CA, USA) for 1 h. For IHC analysis, primary antibodies (anti-KRT5, anti-ΔNp63, and anti-MUC5AC from Abcam; anti-β-catenin and anti-SOX2 from Santa Cruz Biotechnology, Dallas, TX, USA) were applied overnight. After washing with PBS, the sections were treated with a mixture of anti-rabbit and anti-mouse horseradish peroxidase polymer (GBI Labs, Rockville, MD, USA) for 30 min. Diaminobenzidine staining (GBI Labs) was then performed to produce a dark brown color and was followed by counterstaining with hematoxylin.

For IF analysis, sections were incubated overnight with primary anti-ΔNp63 and anti-KRT13 (Santa Cruz Biotechnology) antibodies. After washing, the sections were treated with secondary anti-mouse IgG Alexa Fluor 488 and anti-rabbit IgG Alexa Fluor 647 antibodies (1:1000) from Invitrogen (Waltham, MA, USA), for 2 h. Subsequently, 4′,6-diamidino-2-phenylindole counterstaining (Invitrogen) was performed. The slides were visualized using a confocal laser microscope (LSM 800; Carl Zeiss, Oberkochen, Germany).

2.8. Quantitative and Statistical Analysis

Stained sections were randomly captured from three different fields for analysis under magnifications of 50× for Alcian blue, 200× for H and E and MT staining, and 400× for IHC. To quantify IHC results, we expressed the percentage of positive cells by calculating the proportion of cells with nuclear staining. Specifically, the number of positively stained nuclei was divided by the total number of nuclei in the examined field, and the result was expressed as a percentage to represent the extent of marker expression. Quantitative analysis of pixel values corresponding to the features of interest in each selected area was performed using ImageJ software (64-bit, Java 8 version). Statistical analyses, including unpaired *t*-tests to evaluate differences between groups, were conducted using Prism 8.0 software (GraphPad Software, San Diego, CA, USA). In the calculation of the morphometric index, the sample size was quantified using the sections corresponding to positions IV and V in Figure 1d. Using the measured sample size, the morphometric index was calculated as follows [11,12]:

$$\frac{\text{Free space in nasal cavity}}{\text{Free space in nasal cavity} + \text{Ventral turbinate}} \times 100(\%)$$

3. Results

3.1. Morphological Changes in the Nasal Cavity in the ENS Model

Following turbinoplasty, immediate endoscopic imaging revealed visible tissue damage (Figure 1b). Cross-sectional views of the ventral turbinate taken 56 days post-turbinoplasty showed structural changes suggestive of ENS (Figure 1c). However, even after turbinectomy and observation of the animals for 56 days, the blood biochemistry values remained within the normal range (Table 1). An examination of tissue sections revealed variation in the cross-sectional shape based on the location within the nasal cavity.

Table 1. Hematological parameters.

Variables	Unit	Criterion Range	0 Day	56 Days
CRP	μg/mL	1.5~25.0	2	3
BUN	mg/dL	5.59~18.87	14	6
AST	IU/L	16.4~504	53	29
ALT	IU/L	13.2~53.2	50	51

In the ENS model, increased fibrosis resulting from the defect damage narrowed the nasal cavity anteriorly, and the nasal cavity was widened beyond the defect, as observed in the tissue sections (Figure 1d,e). The ventral turbinate volume decreased significantly to 23.44%± 8.29% in the ENS model relative to the control. Furthermore, the morphometric index was 91.30% ± 4.73% in the ENS group compared to 60.02% ± 9.20% in the control, indicating significant expansion of the nasal cavity (Figure 1f).

3.2. Histological Changes in the Mucosal Epithelium in the ENS Model

To evaluate histological changes in the ENS model, ciliary coverage was examined. Observations revealed the absence of cilia and the presence of bacilli (Figure 2a,b). H and E staining of cross-sectioned tissues showed squamous metaplasia in the ENS model (Figure 3a), in which columnar epithelium transitioned into stratified squamous epithelium (Figure 3b). Additionally, overexpression of the basal-cell markers KRT5 and ΔNp63 suggested a shift in cell composition, with levels increasing from 47.22% ± 5.9% to 75.57% ± 3.40% and from 2.66% ± 1.33% to 49.92% ± 7.0%, respectively. Co-expression of ΔNp63 and KRT13 confirmed the presence of squamous cells in the ENS model (Figure 4a). The expression levels of β-catenin and SOX2 were significantly elevated, from 1.77% ± 0.54% to 77.51% ± 3.64% and from 0.82% ± 0.45% to 78.98% ± 7.19%, respectively, suggesting their involvement in driving squamous metaplasia in the ENS model (Figure 4b,c).

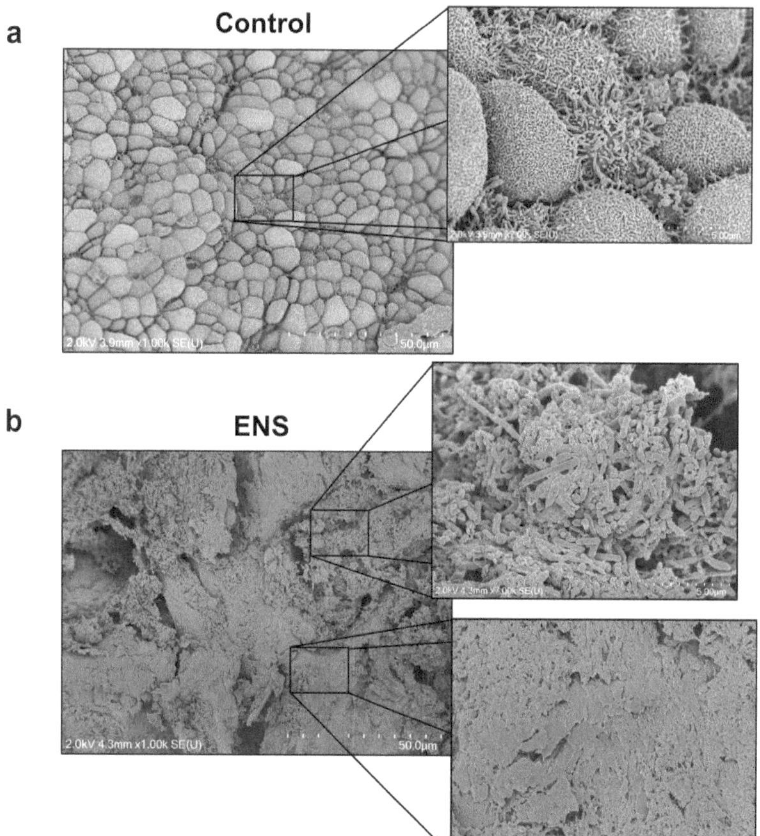

Figure 2. Surface changes in the ventral turbinate in the ENS model. (**a**,**b**) Surface images of the ventral turbinate captured by scanning electron microscopy at magnifications of 1000× and 7000×.

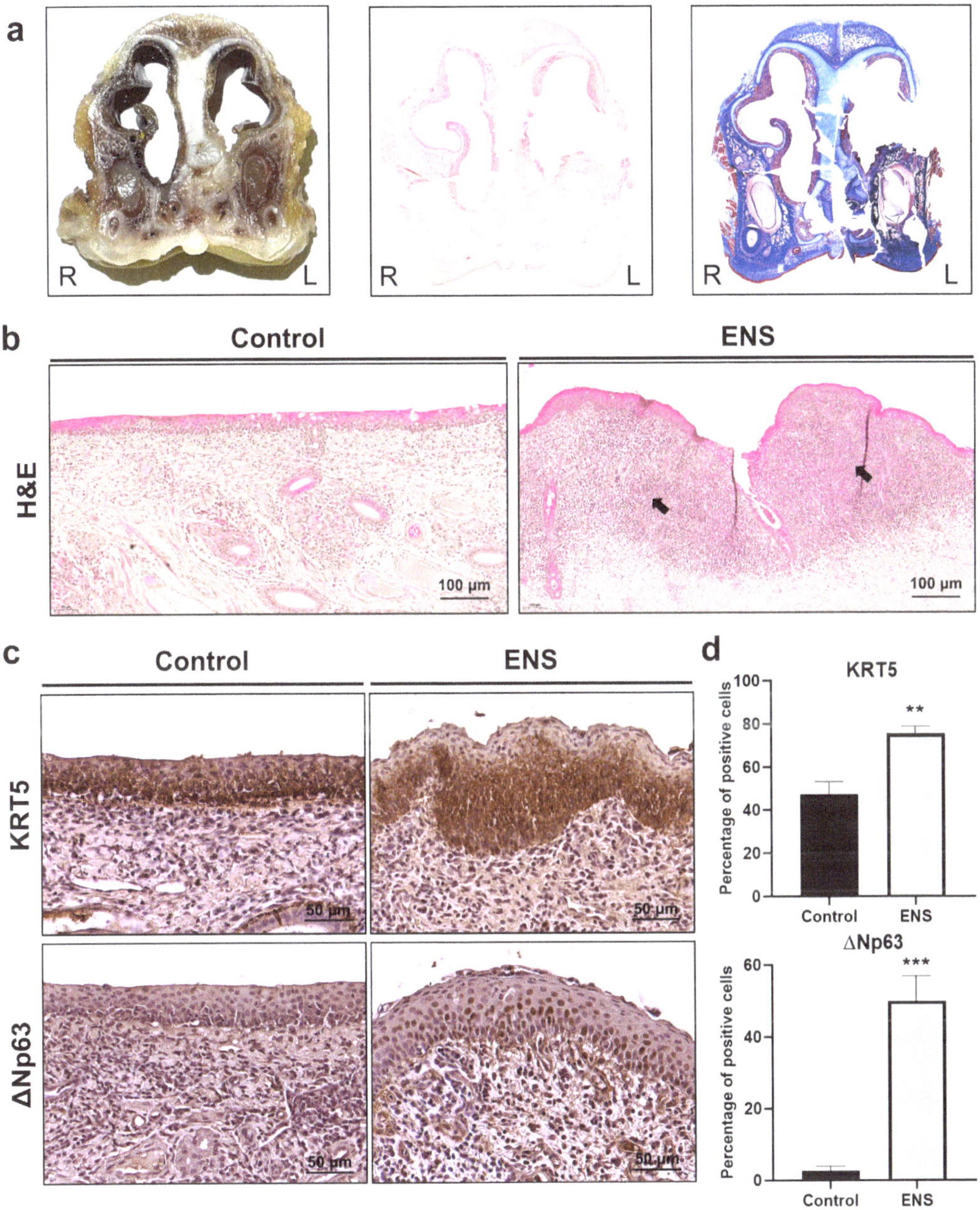

Figure 3. Histological alterations in the epithelium in the ENS model. (**a**) Cross-sectional images of tissue samples with H and E and MT staining. (**b**) Tissues were examined at 200× magnification following H and E staining to compare histological features between the control and ENS groups. Arrow indicates squamous cell metaplasia. (**c**) IHC staining for KRT5 and ΔNp63, examined at 400× magnification. (**d**) IHC images were compared quantitatively; data are means ± SD (** $p < 0.01$, *** $p < 0.001$).

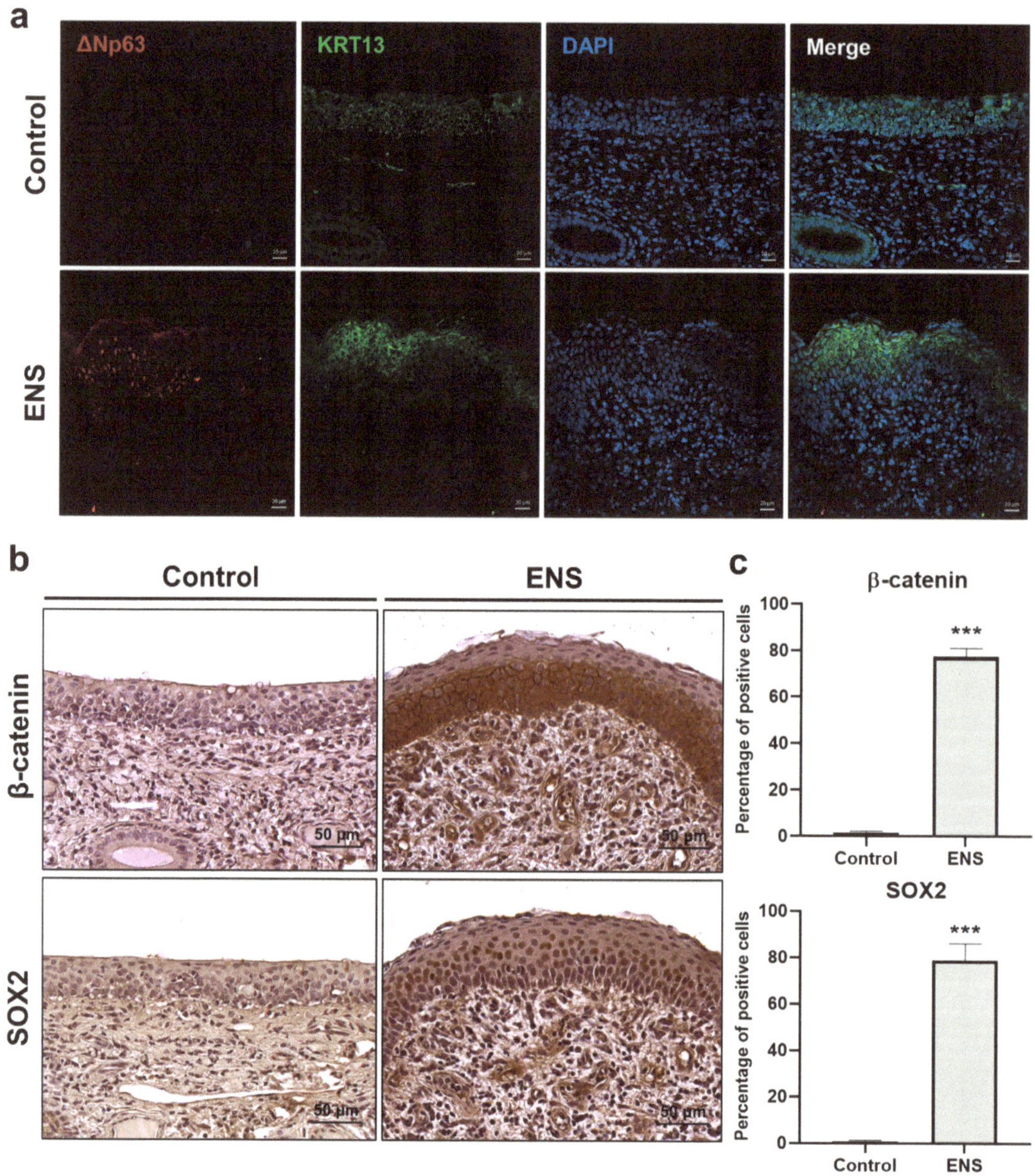

Figure 4. The difference in protein expression in ENS squamous epithelium. (**a**) Comparison of ΔNp63 and KRT13 co-expression between the two groups using IF staining. (**b**) IHC images of β-catenin and SOX2. (**c**) Percentages of stained cells in the epithelium; data are means ± SD (*** $p < 0.001$).

Images of H and E-stained tissues showed an increase in the number of cells with goblet cell morphology in the pseudostratified epithelium (Figure 5a). Subsequent Alcian blue staining to assess mucin expression revealed an increase from 7.12% to 21.51% (Figure 5b,c). Moreover, there was a significant increase in number of MUC5AC-positive cells in the goblet metaplasia area, from 13.33 ± 2.52 to 94.0 ± 44.4, indicating a marked increase in MUC5AC expression (Figure 5d,e).

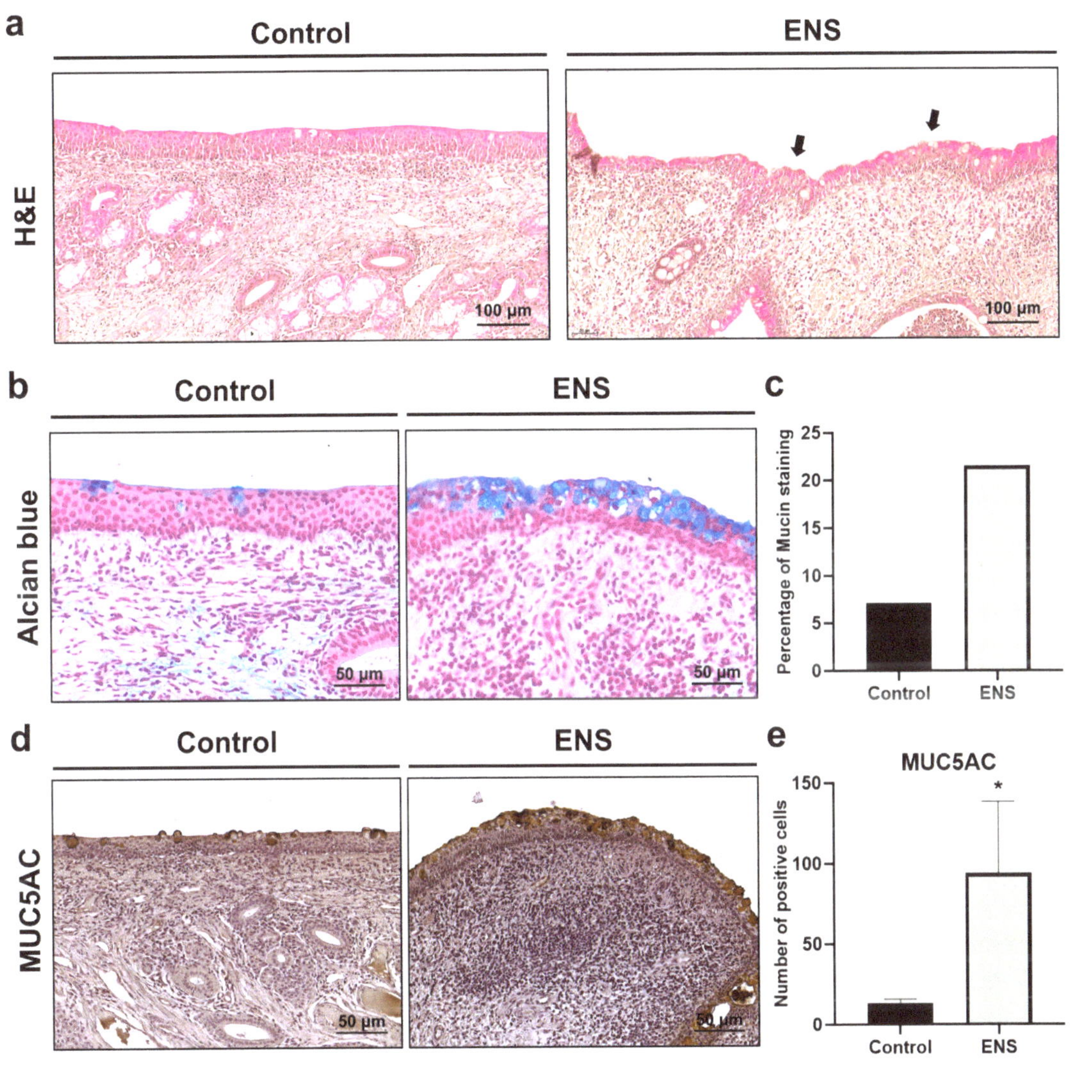

Figure 5. Goblet cell metaplasia was observed in the ENS epithelium. (**a**) Goblet cell metaplasia (arrows) was observed at 200× magnification following H and E staining. (**b**,**c**) Mucin were visualized following Alcian blue staining and plotted as percentages. (**d**,**e**) Goblet cell metaplasia was visualized using IHC with MUC5AC at 400× magnification and plotted as numbers of stained cells; data are means ± SD (* $p < 0.05$).

3.3. Histological Modifications in Submucosal Structure in the ENS Model

Submucosal fibrosis and glandular atrophy were confirmed through H and E staining (Figure 6a). Further assessment of fibrosis using MT staining showed an increase in blue-stained collagen within the submucosa (Figure 6b). The collagen-stained area as a percentage of the submucosal area increased two-fold, from 25.46% in the control to 50.89% ± 6.83% in the ENS model (Figure 6c). Additionally, H and E staining revealed a marked decrease in the size of the submucosal glands (Figure 6d) from 100.0% in the control to 4.38% ± 5.51% in the ENS model (Figure 6e).

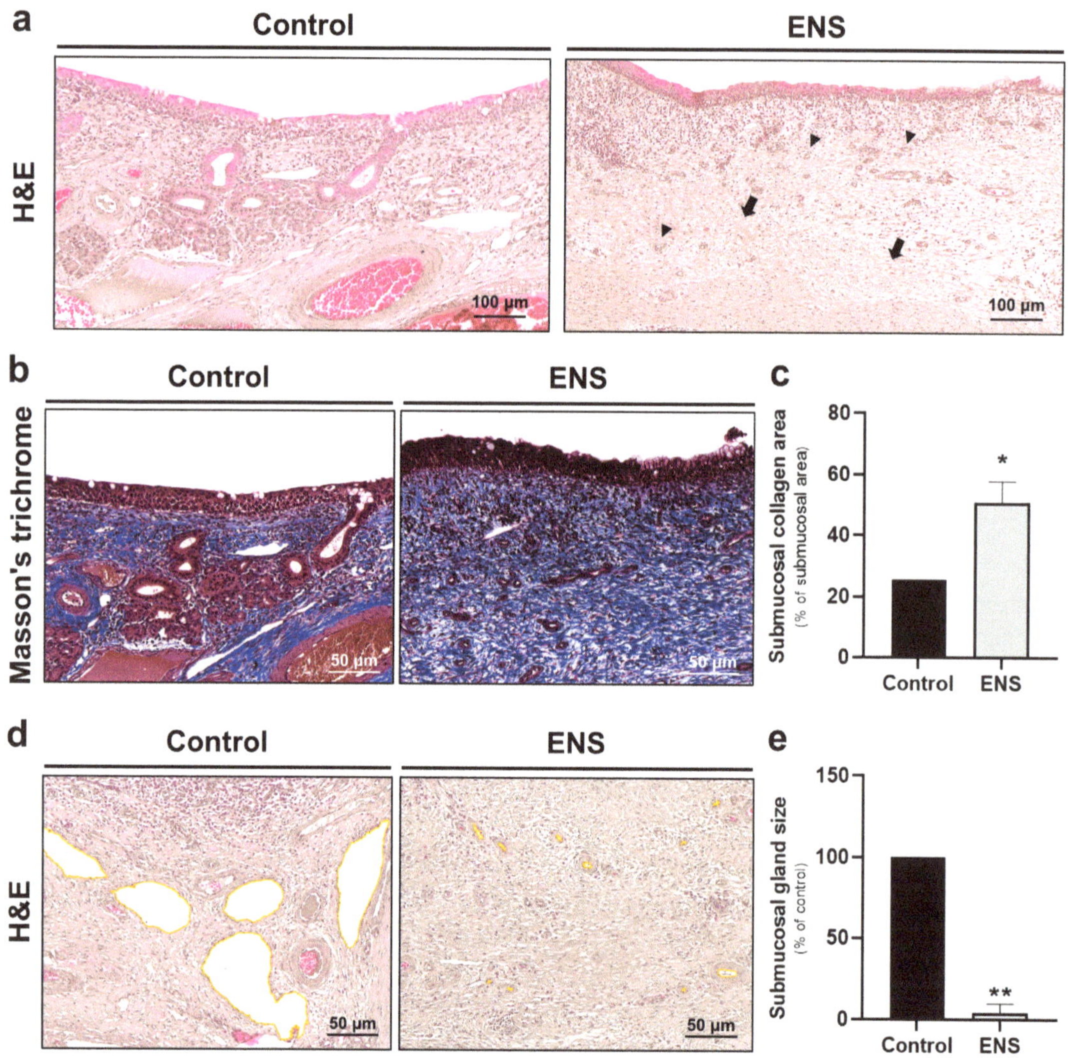

Figure 6. Histological changes were observed in ENS submucosa. (**a**) Histological changes in the submucosa were observed at 200× magnification following H and E staining. Arrows and arrowheads indicate submucosal fibrosis and glandular atrophy, respectively. (**b**,**c**) Collagen distributions in the submucosa were visualized using MT staining and plotted as means ± SD. (**d**,**e**) Submucosal glands (yellow lines) were visualized at 200× magnification following H and E staining, and their sizes were plotted as means ± SD (* $p < 0.05$, ** $p < 0.01$).

4. Discussion

Surgical removal of the nasal turbinate can disrupt nasal function, potentially triggering the onset of ENS, which typically occurs after inferior turbinate resection, with a lower chance of occurrence following middle turbinate resection [13,14]. Therefore, it is necessary to identify animals in which ENS can be induced through turbinoplasty while the inferior turbinate is visualized with an endoscope. We hypothesized that animals in which atrophic rhinitis (AR) can be induced could be suitable for the induction of ENS. Atrophic rhinitis models have been developed using swine and rats, with the condition induced by toxins from *Pasteurella multocida or Bordetella bronchiseptica* [15,16]. These models differ from the model developed in the present study because they involve primary AR induced using bacterial strains and not secondary AR caused by nasal surgery. However, turbinectomy/turbinoplasty can be performed in swine using the same procedure as in humans, so we attempted to create a swine ENS model and observed whether it could replicate key characteristics seen in human patients with ENS.

In our swine model, following turbinoplasty, we observed a reduction in ventral turbinate volume. This is reminiscent of the AR induced in swine models, where atrophy of the nasal turbinates leads to an expansion of the nasal cavity's free space. As a result, the morphometric index increased, reflecting the degree of turbinate atrophy and associated structural changes [17,18]. In animals infected with bacteria such as *Pasteurella multocida* or *Bordetella bronchiseptica*, hematological parameters such as CRP, BUN, AST and ALT showed increases [19–21]. However, in our study, these parameters did not show a significant increase. Instead, we observed morphological changes in the nasal cavity. This suggests that the observed changes in our model may not be attributable to bacterial infection, indicating the possibility that other factors might be responsible for these structural alterations.

In humans, these histological changes include squamous and goblet cell metaplasia in the mucosal epithelium and fibrosis and gland atrophy in the submucosa. Furthermore, keratinization is observed in some areas where squamous cell metaplasia has occurred [22,23]. In our swine ENS model, the normal respiratory columnar epithelium was transformed into stratified squamous epithelium and keratinization was observed in some areas, along with squamous cell metaplasia. This indicates that our model has the potential to effectively replicate these histological changes.

The TP63, KRT5, KRT13, and KRT15 genes are canonical markers of squamous epithelial cells, although TP63 and KRT5 are also widely recognized as canonical basal-cell markers in the airway epithelium, imposing limitations when they are used alone to identify squamous epithelial cells [24]. In a study using single-cell sequencing analysis to categorize airway basal cells into clusters, the basal cell markers TP63 and KRT5 were expressed throughout the clusters, whereas KRT13 was specifically expressed in the basal–squamous cluster [25]. The TP63 gene has two main isoforms: one retaining (TA) and the other lacking (ΔN) the transactivation domain [26]. ΔNp63 plays a role in epithelial morphogenesis, where its expression and activity are pivotal in transcriptional and post-transcriptional processes during squamous differentiation. It is predominantly expressed in stratified squamous epithelium, where it is particularly localized to the basal cell layer [27–29]. In the ENS model, we observed co-expression of KRT5 and KRT13, as well as overexpression of ΔNp63. This suggests that our ENS model not only replicates the histological characteristics of squamous cell metaplasia but could also have the potential to mimic its associated biomarkers.

The Wnt/β–catenin signaling pathway regulates squamous differentiation in airway basal cells [30,31]. There is a reciprocal relationship between levels of expression of the ΔNp63 gene and the Wnt/β–catenin signaling pathway. ΔNp63 can upregulate the expression of Frizzled, a Wnt ligand receptor, and the Wnt/β–catenin signaling pathway acts as an upstream regulator of ΔNp63 [32,33]. The SOX2 gene plays a crucial role in both the development and the maintenance of squamous epithelium, interacting with ΔNp63 [34]. In our ENS model, we observed significant increases in β-catenin and SOX2 expression. These two signals have co-relationships with ΔNp63. However, further research is needed to determine which gene is activated first and then influences the other during the pathogenesis of ENS.

The ENS model exhibited a significant increase in mucin expression, particularly in goblet cells. This finding aligns with the histological shift from ciliated cells to goblet cells, along with the confirmed MUC5AC expression in areas with goblet metaplasia.

Interestingly, research has suggested that 35% of patients with ENS experience squamous and goblet cell metaplasia simultaneously [12,35].

Submucosal fibrosis was observed through the visualization of collagen fibers associated with the high collagen concentrations in fibrotic cells. The collagen-fiber area was doubled in the ENS model, although the collagen area was also high in the control. The swine vomeronasal organ consists of connective tissue containing collagen and elastin, resulting in high expression of collagen [36]. Moreover, a significant decrease in the size of the submucosal gland was evident, likely due to the progression of submucosal fibrosis, which may have further affected atrophic changes of the nasal mucosa. The resulting glandular atrophy leads to dryness in the nasal cavity and the formation of dried crusts. Moreover, the absence of cilia impedes the clearance of secretions, further facilitating crust formation [37].

We developed an ENS model by simulating the turbinoplasty performed in humans. Since the surgical techniques used in human procedures require experimentation on large animals, swine were selected for this study. However, in a difference from the human nasal structure, swine possess a protruding snout, which results in anatomical differences [38–41]. The effect of these anatomical discrepancies on the development of the model remains unclear. Furthermore, one of the tools for diagnosis of ENS in humans, the Empty Nose Syndrome 6-Item Questionnaire, assesses subjective symptoms such as dryness, nasal crusting, nasal burning, lack of air sensation, suffocation, and the sensation of the nose being too open [42,43]. These patient-reported outcomes are challenging to evaluate in swine. Therefore, there is a need to develop alternative diagnostic methods that can address these limitations in animal models.

5. Conclusions

As we noted, turbinoplasty can be performed in the swine model in a way similar to how it is performed in humans. This model may be helpful for evaluating the various surgical or mucosal regenerative approaches being developed to treat ENS. Additionally, our swine model expressed markers that are also found in ENS patients, which will provide further information on the appropriateness of the model and treatment effectiveness.

Author Contributions: Conceptualization, D.H.K. and S.W.K.; Methodology, D.B.P. and D.W.J.; Software, D.B.P. and D.W.J.; Validation, D.H.K. and S.W.K.; Formal analysis, D.B.P.; Investigation, D.B.P. and D.W.J.; Resources, D.W.J.; Data curation, D.B.P.; Writing—original draft, D.B.P.; Writing—review & editing, D.B.P., D.W.J., D.H.K. and S.W.K.; Supervision, D.W.J., D.H.K. and S.W.K.; Project administration, D.H.K. and S.W.K.; Funding acquisition, D.H.K. All authors have read and agreed to the published version of the manuscript.

Funding: This work was supported by the National Research Foundation of Korea (NRF; grant no. RS-2023-00209494 and 22021M3F7A1083232), and the Korean Fund for Regenerative Medicine (grant no. 23C0121L1).

Institutional Review Board Statement: All animals involved in this experiment were cared for following the ethical standards. All procedures were conducted in compliance with applicable ethical standards and received approval from the Institutional Animal Care and Use Committee of CRONEX (CRONEX-IACUC Approval No. 202309-002 and Approval Date 8 September 2023).

Informed Consent Statement: Not applicable.

Data Availability Statement: The data analyzed in this study are available from the corresponding author upon reasonable request.

Acknowledgments: The authors express their gratitude to the Catholic Medical Center Research Foundation for financial support provided in the 2023 program year.

Conflicts of Interest: The authors declare that they have no competing interests, financial or otherwise, that could influence the work reported in this manuscript.

Abbreviations

Empty nose syndrome; ENS, Atrophic rhinitis; AR, Institutional Animal Care and Use Committee; IACUC, Scanning Electron Microscopy; SEM, Phosphate-buffered saline; PBS, Hematoxylin and Eosin; H & E, Masson's trichrome; MT, Immunohistochemistry; IHC, Immunofluorescence; IF, immunofluorescence.

References

1. Moore, E.J.; Kern, E.B. Atrophic rhinitis: A review of 242 cases. *Am. J. Rhinol.* **2001**, *15*, 355–361. [CrossRef] [PubMed]
2. Chhabra, N.; Houser, S.M. The diagnosis and management of empty nose syndrome. *Otolaryngol. Clin. North Am.* **2009**, *42*, 311–330. [CrossRef] [PubMed]
3. Shah, K.; Guarderas, J.; Krishnaswamy, G. Empty nose syndrome and atrophic rhinitis. *Ann. Allergy Asthma Immunol.* **2016**, *117*, 217–220. [CrossRef] [PubMed]
4. Gunaratne, D.A.; Thamboo, A.V. Empty Nose Syndrome as an Iatrogenic Condition from Surgery. *Curr. Otorhinolaryngol. Rep.* **2023**, *11*, 458–465. [CrossRef]
5. Fu, C.H.; Chen, C.C.; Huang, C.C.; Chang, P.H.; Chen, Y.W.; Tang, Y.C.; Lee, T.J. Morphology, Not Only Volume: A Study on Empty Nose Syndrome and Inferior Turbinates. *Laryngoscope* **2024**, *134*, 3060–3066. [CrossRef]
6. Kuan, E.C.; Suh, J.D.; Wang, M.B. Empty nose syndrome. *Curr. Allergy Asthma Rep.* **2015**, *15*, 493. [CrossRef]
7. Talmadge, J.; Nayak, J.V.; Yao, W.; Citardi, M.J. Management of Postsurgical Empty Nose Syndrome. *Facial Plast. Surg. Clin. North Am.* **2019**, *27*, 465–475. [CrossRef]
8. Leong, S.C. The clinical efficacy of surgical interventions for empty nose syndrome: A systematic review. *Laryngoscope* **2015**, *125*, 1557–1562. [CrossRef]
9. Życzko, K.; Sielawa, H.; Łaszyn, M. Serum C-reactive protein (CRP) levels and the values of blood hematological indices in piglets. *Sci. Ann. Pol. Soc. Anim. Prod.* **2012**, *8*, 63–71.
10. Yeom, S.C.; Cho, S.Y.; Park, C.G.; Lee, W.J. Analysis of reference interval and age-related changes in serum biochemistry and hematology in the specific pathogen free miniature pig. *Lab. Anim. Res.* **2012**, *28*, 245–253. [CrossRef]
11. Hamilton, T.D.; Roe, J.M.; Webster, A.J. Synergistic role of gaseous ammonia in etiology of *Pasteurella multocida*-induced atrophic rhinitis in swine. *J. Clin. Microbiol.* **1996**, *34*, 2185–2190. [CrossRef] [PubMed]
12. Sumaily, I.A.; Hakami, N.A.; Almutairi, A.D.; Alsudays, A.A.; Abulqusim, E.M.; Abualgasem, M.M.; Alghulikah, A.A.; Alserhani, A.A. An Updated Review on Atrophic Rhinitis and Empty Nose Syndrome. *Ear Nose Throat J.* **2023**, *14*, 1455613231185022. [CrossRef] [PubMed]
13. Scheithauer, M.O. Surgery of the turbinates and "empty nose" syndrome. *GMS Curr. Top. Otorhinolaryngol. Head Neck Surg.* **2011**, *9*, 98–126. [CrossRef]
14. Law, R.H.; Ahmed, A.M.; Van Harn, M.; Craig, J.R. Middle turbinate resection is unlikely to cause empty nose syndrome in first year postoperatively. *Am. J. Otolaryngol.* **2021**, *42*, 102931. [CrossRef] [PubMed]
15. Horiguchi, Y. Swine atrophic rhinitis caused by *pasteurella multocida* toxin and *bordetella* dermonecrotic toxin. *Curr. Top. Microbiol. Immunol.* **2012**, *361*, 113–129. [CrossRef] [PubMed]
16. Balur, M.B.; Kocak, H.E.; Altinay, S.; Ozdamar, K.; Taskin, U.; Oktay, M.F. Is submucosal fat injection effective in atrophic rhinitis? An experimental animal study. *Eur. Arch. Otorhinolaryngol.* **2017**, *274*, 3637–3642. [CrossRef]
17. Hamilton, T.D.C.; Roe, J.M.; Hayes, C.M.; Jones, P.; Pearson, G.R.; Webster, A.J.F. Contributory and Exacerbating Roles of Gaseous Ammonia and Organic Dust in the Etiology of Atrophic Rhinitis. *Clin. Diagn. Lab. Immunol.* **1999**, *6*, 199–203. [CrossRef]
18. Magyar, T.; Donkó, T.; Repa, I.; Kovács, M. Regeneration of toxigenic *Pasteurella multocida* induced severe turbinate atrophy in pigs detected by computed tomography. *BMC Vet. Res.* **2013**, *9*, 222. [CrossRef]
19. Allam, T.S.; Said, L.; Elsayed, M.S.A.E.; Saleh, N. Clinical Investigation of the Pathogenicity of *Pasteurella multocida* Isolated from Cattle in Egypt Regarding its Effect on Hematological, Biochemical, and Oxidant-Antioxidant Biomarkers as well as Proinflammatory Cytokines and Acute Phase Proteins. *Adv. Anim. Vet. Sci.* **2021**, *9*, 792–801. [CrossRef]
20. Thakor, J.C.; Kumar, P.; Dinesh, M.; Vishwa, K.V.; Qureshi, S.; Singh, K.P.; Sahoo, M. Sequential development of pathology and pathogenesis of capsular serotype D of *Pasteurella multocida* of porcine origin in mouse model. *Indian J. Vet. Pathol.* **2020**, *44*, 69–80. [CrossRef]
21. Canonne, A.M.; Menard, M.; Maurey, C.; Benchrekroun, G.; Fernandes Rodrigues, N.; Billen, F.; Clercx, C. Comparison of C-reactive protein concentrations in dogs with *Bordetella bronchiseptica* infection and aspiration bronchopneumonia. *J. Vet. Intern. Med.* **2021**, *35*, 1519–1524. [CrossRef] [PubMed]
22. Gordiienko, I.M.; Gubar, O.S.; Sulik, R.; Kunakh, T.; Zlatskiy, I.; Zlatska, A. Empty nose syndrome pathogenesis and cell-based biotechnology products as a new option for treatment. *World J. Stem. Cells* **2021**, *13*, 1293–1306. [CrossRef] [PubMed]
23. Dzhenkov, D.L.; Stoyanov, G.S.; Georgiev, R.; Sapundzhiev, N. Histopathological Findings in an Unclassifiable Case of Empty Nose Syndrome with Long-term Follow-up. *Cureus* **2018**, *10*, e2655. [CrossRef] [PubMed]
24. Stavniichuk, R.; DeLaForest, A.; Thompson, C.A.; Miller, J.; Souza, R.F.; Battle, M.A. GATA4 blocks squamous epithelial cell gene expression in human esophageal squamous cells. *Sci. Rep.* **2021**, *11*, 3206. [CrossRef] [PubMed]
25. Zhou, Y.; Yang, Y.; Guo, L.; Qian, J.; Ge, J.; Sinner, D.; Ding, H.; Califano, A.; Cardoso, W.V. Airway basal cells show regionally distinct potential to undergo metaplastic differentiation. *eLife* **2022**, *11*, e80083. [CrossRef]

26. Mitani, Y.; Li, J.; Weber, R.S.; Lippman, S.L.; Flores, E.R.; Caulin, C.; El-Naggar, A.K. Expression and regulation of the DeltaN and TAp63 isoforms in salivary gland tumorigenesis clinical and experimental findings. *Am. J. Pathol.* **2011**, *179*, 391–399. [CrossRef]
27. Samanta, A.; Saha, P.; Johnson, O.; Bishayee, A.; Sinha, D. Dysregulation of delta Np63 alpha in squamous cell carcinoma and its therapeutic targeting. *Biochim. Biophy.s Acta Rev. Cancer* **2024**, *1879*, 189034. [CrossRef]
28. Moses, M.A.; George, A.L.; Sakakibara, N.; Mahmood, K.; Ponnamperuma, R.M.; King, K.E.; Weinberg, W.C. Molecular Mechanisms of p63-Mediated Squamous Cancer Pathogenesis. *Int. J. Mol. Sci.* **2019**, *20*, 3590. [CrossRef]
29. Gatti, V.; Fierro, C.; Annicchiarico-Petruzzelli, M.; Melino, G.; Peschiaroli, A. ΔNp63 in squamous cell carcinoma: Defining the oncogenic routes affecting epigenetic landscape and tumour microenvironment. *Mol. Oncol.* **2019**, *13*, 981–1001. [CrossRef]
30. McCravy, M.S.; Ingram, J.L. A Hint from Wnt: Squamous Cell Differentiation in the Airways. *Am. J. Respir. Cell. Mol. Biol.* **2023**, *68*, 601–602. [CrossRef]
31. Zhang, Y.; Black, K.E.; Phung, T.N.; Thundivalappil, S.R.; Lin, T.; Wang, W.; Xu, J.; Zhang, C.; Hariri, L.P.; Lapey, A.; et al. Human Airway Basal Cells Undergo Reversible Squamous Differentiation and Reshape Innate Immunity. *Am. J. Respir. Cell. Mol. Biol.* **2023**, *68*, 664–678. [CrossRef] [PubMed]
32. Xu, Y.; Yang, X.; Xiong, Q.; Han, J.; Zhu, Q. The dual role of p63 in cancer. *Front. Oncol.* **2023**, *13*, 1116061. [CrossRef] [PubMed]
33. Li, Y.; Giovannini, S.; Wang, T.; Fang, J.; Li, P.; Shao, C.; Wang, Y.; Shi, Y.; Candi, E.; TOR centre; et al. p63: A crucial player in epithelial stemness regulation. *Oncogene* **2023**, *42*, 3371–3384. [CrossRef] [PubMed]
34. Watanabe, H.; Ma, Q.; Peng, S.; Adelmant, G.; Swain, D.; Song, W.; Fox, C.; Francis, J.M.; Pedamallu, C.S.; DeLuca, D.S.; et al. SOX2 and p63 colocalize at genetic loci in squamous cell carcinomas. *J. Clin. Investig.* **2014**, *124*, 1636–1645. [CrossRef] [PubMed]
35. Wu, C.L.; Fu, C.H.; Lee, T.J. Distinct Histopathology Characteristics in Empty Nose Syndrome. *Laryngoscope* **2021**, *131*, E14–E18. [CrossRef]
36. Salazar, I.; Lombardero, M.; Cifuentes, J.M.; Sanchez Quinteiro, P.; Aleman, N. Morphogenesis and growth of the soft tissue and cartilage of the vomeronasal organ in pigs. *J. Anat.* **2003**, *202*, 503–514. [CrossRef]
37. Beard, S. Rhinitis. *Prim. Care* **2014**, *41*, 33–46. [CrossRef]
38. Orhan, M.; Govsa, F.; Saylam, C. A surgical view of the superior nasal turbinate: Anatomical study. *Eur. Arch. Otorhinolaryngol.* **2010**, *267*, 909–916. [CrossRef]
39. Jing, J.Y.; Lei, D.; Qing, H.Y.; Qian, Y. Histological and anatomical structure of the nasal cavity of Bama minipigs. *PLoS ONE* **2017**, *12*, e0173902. [CrossRef]
40. Marks, T.N.; Maddux, S.D.; Butaric, L.N.; Franciscus, R.G. Climatic adaptation in human inferior nasal turbinate morphology: Evidence from Arctic and equatorial populations. *Am. J. Phys. Anthropol.* **2019**, *169*, 498–512. [CrossRef]
41. Yuk, J.; Akash, M.M.H.; Chakraborty, A.; Basu, S.; Chamorro, L.P.; Jung, S. Morphology of pig nasal structure and modulation of airflow and basic thermal conditioning. *Integr. Comp. Biol.* **2023**, *63*, 304–314. [CrossRef] [PubMed]
42. Velasquez, N.; Thamboo, A.; Habib, A.R.; Huang, Z.; Nayak, J.V. The Empty Nose Syndrome 6-Item Questionnaire (ENS6Q): A validated 6-item questionnaire as a diagnostic aid for empty nose syndrome patients. *Int. Forum Allergy Rhinol.* **2017**, *7*, 64–71. [CrossRef] [PubMed]
43. Huang, C.C.; Wu, P.W.; Lee, C.C.; Huang, C.C.; Fu, C.H.; Chang, P.H.; Lee, T.J. Comparison of SNOT-25 and ENS6Q in evaluating patients with empty nose syndrome. *Laryngoscope Investig. Otolaryngol.* **2022**, *7*, 342–348. [CrossRef] [PubMed]

medicina

MDPI

Article

$PM_{2.5}$ Induces Pyroptosis via Activation of the ROS/NF-κB Signaling Pathway in Bronchial Epithelial Cells

Ji-Young Kang [1], Hyunsu Choi [2], Jeong-Min Oh [2], Minsu Kim [3] and Dong-Chang Lee [3,*]

[1] Division of Pulmonary, Allergy, and Critical Care Medicine, Department of Internal Medicine, Jeju National University Hospital, 15 Aran 13-gil, Jeju-si 63241, Republic of Korea; rkdwldud4221@gmail.com
[2] Clinical Research Institute, Daejeon St. Mary's Hospital, Daeheung-dong, Jung-gu, Daejeon 34943, Republic of Korea; 20110201@cmcnu.or.kr (H.C.); yejmdh@cmcnu.or.kr (J.-M.O.)
[3] Department of Otorhinolaryngology-Head and Neck Surgery, Daejeon St. Mary's Hospital, College of Medicine, The Catholic University of Korea, 64 Daeheung-ro, Jung-gu, Daejeon 34943, Republic of Korea; tokimminsu@gmail.com
* Correspondence: sayman@hanmail.net; Tel.: +82-42-220-9266; Fax: +82-42-221-9580

Abstract: *Background and Objectives*: Fine particulate matter, $PM_{2.5}$, is becoming a major threat to human health, particularly in terms of respiratory diseases. Pyroptosis is a recently discovered and distinct form of cell death, characterized by pore formation in the cell membrane and secretions of proinflammatory cytokines. There has been little research on the effect of $PM_{2.5}$ on pyroptosis, especially in airway epithelium. We investigated whether $PM_{2.5}$-related oxidative stress induces pyroptosis in bronchial epithelial cells and defined the underlying mechanisms. *Materials and Methods*: After exposure of a BEAS-2B cell line to $PM_{2.5}$ concentration of 20 μg/mL, reactive oxygen species (ROS) levels, parameters related to pyroptosis, and NF-κB signaling were measured by Western blotting, immunofluorescence, and ELISA (Enzyme-linked immunosorbent assay). *Results*: $PM_{2.5}$ induced pyroptotic cell death, accompanied by LDH (Lactate dehydrogenase) release and increased uptake of propidium iodide in a dose-dependent manner. $PM_{2.5}$ activated the NLRP3-casp1-gasdermin D pathway, with resulting secretions of the proinflammatory cytokines IL-1β and IL-18. The pyroptosis activated by $PM_{2.5}$ was alleviated significantly by NLRP3 inhibitor. In $PM_{2.5}$-exposed BEAS-2B cells, levels of intracellular ROS and NF-κB p65 increased. ROS scavenger inhibited the expression of the NLRP3 inflammasome, and the NF-κB inhibitor attenuated pyroptotic cell death triggered by $PM_{2.5}$ exposure, indicating that the ROS/NF-κB pathway is involved in $PM_{2.5}$-induced pyroptosis. *Conclusions*: These findings show that $PM_{2.5}$ exposure can cause cell injury by NLRP3-inflammasome-mediated pyroptosis by upregulating the ROS/NF-κB pathway in airway epithelium.

Keywords: particulate matter 2.5; reactive oxygen species; pyroptosis; respiratory epithelium; NF-kappa B

1. Introduction

Particulate matter (PM), a major air pollutant, is becoming a global public health concern. Defined by its aerodynamic diameter, $PM_{2.5}$ ($\leq$2.5 μm diameter)—often called fine particulate matter—is the particle size class with the most detrimental effects on the human body. $PM_{2.5}$ has peculiar characteristics such as a large surface area; its adsorbed substances including polycyclic aromatic hydrocarbon, heavy metals, and microbes; and its easy transportation to the upper and lower respiratory tract as well as other systemic organs [1,2]. Cardiovascular diseases such as ischemic heart disease and stroke, respiratory diseases, lung cancer, type 2 diabetes mellitus, and preterm birth are the five most common conditions that can be attributed to $PM_{2.5}$ exposure [3–7]. In 2019, there were an estimated 4.15 million ambient $PM_{2.5}$-related deaths globally, a remarkable increase of 102% from 1990 to 2019 [8,9].

Previous research has shown that $PM_{2.5}$-induced tissue damage primarily in the respiratory tract through oxidative stress, proinflammatory responses, cytotoxicity, apoptosis, and DNA damage [10–14]. In particular, reactive oxygen species (ROS), which are byproducts of oxidative stress, have adverse health effects on chronic obstructive lung disease (COPD), pulmonary fibrosis, and pulmonary infections through various mechanisms such as oxidization of DNA and lipids, TGF- β (transforming growth factor-beta) signaling activation, and epithelial barrier disruption [15–17]. We previously demonstrated that exposure to $PM_{2.5}$ induces proinflammatory signaling activation and tight junction dysfunction via ROS generation in airway epithelial cell lines [14,18].

Pyroptosis is a newly discovered form of programmed cell death, which is executed by the gasdermin (GSDM) protein family and mediated by the inflammasome pathway [19]. Through pore formation in the cell membrane and release of the proinflammatory cytokines IL (interleukin)-1β and IL-18, pyroptosis not only eliminates harmful microbes from the body but also aggravates inflammatory conditions including respiratory diseases such as asthma or COPD [20]. Some research has shown that foreign insults such as allergens, viral infections, or cigarette smoke induce pyroptosis via the NLRP3 inflammasome signaling pathway in bronchial epithelial cells, resulting in persistent inflammation and/or airway remodeling [21–23]. However, few studies have examined the association between $PM_{2.5}$ and pyroptosis, particularly in airway epithelium. This study aimed to investigate the effect of $PM_{2.5}$ in human bronchial epithelial cells as a first-contact physiological barrier to noxious stimuli, as well as to elucidate the underlying mechanisms with a focus on NLRP3-inflammasome-induced pyroptosis with ROS involvement.

2. Materials and Methods

2.1. Chemical Reagents

Bronchial epithelial growth medium (BEGM) was obtained from Lonza (Walkersville, MD, USA). Antibiotic–antimycotic solution was purchased from Gibco (Thermo Fisher Scientific, Waltham, MA, USA). $PM_{2.5}$ (NIST SRM 1650b), ROS scavenger N-acetylcysteine (NAC), NLRP3 Inhibitor MCC950, NF-κB inhibitor BAY 11-7082, and propidium iodide (PI) were purchased from Millipore Sigma (Saint Louis, MO, USA). The fluorescent stains 4,6-diamidino-2-phenylindole (DAPI) and 2,7-dichlorodihydrofluorescein diacetate (DCFH-DA) were obtained from Invitrogen (Carlsbad, CA, USA). The cell viability reagent, 3-(4,5-dimethylthiazol-2-yl)-2,5-dipehnlytetrazolium bromide, was from DoGen (Seoul, Korea). Antibodies against NOD-like receptor protein-3 (NLRP3), cleaved N-terminal gasdermin D (GSDMD-N), nuclear factor (NF)-κB p65, 3-glyceraldehyde phosphate dehydrogenase (GAPDH), and lamin-B1 were from Cell Signaling Technology (Danvers, MA, USA). The cleaved form of caspase-1 (Casp1) was from Santa Cruz Biotechnology (Santa Cruz, CA, USA).

2.2. Cell Culture and $PM_{2.5}$ Exposure

The human bronchial epithelial cell line BEAS-2B was obtained from the American Type Culture Collection (Manassas, VA, USA). The cells were grown in culture dishes at 37 °C in 5% CO_2 using BEGM medium containing all the recommended supplements (Lonza). The culture medium was replaced every two days. Cells were plated at 70–80% confluence and used the next day. A stock solution of $PM_{2.5}$ at a concentration of 50 mg/mL was prepared in PBS and subsequently diluted to the desired concentrations, 10, 20, and 40 μg/mL in the culture medium.

2.3. Cell Viability Measurement and Lactate Dehydrogenase (LDH) Release Assay

After the cells were treated with $PM_{2.5}$ at different concentrations, 0, 10, 20, and 40 μg/mL for 24 h, the culture medium was collected and centrifuged at 300 g for 5 min to precipitate suspended cells. The supernatants were stored at −80 °C until further analysis. Viability of the precipitated cells was measured after adding 3-(4,5-dimethylthiazol-2-yl)-2,5-diphenlytetrazolium bromide as a solution and incubating the cells for 2 h. Absorbance was recorded at 450 nm in a microplate reader (Bio-Rad, Hercules, CA, USA). As for cytotoxicity, LDH levels in the supernatants were determined using an LDH Cytotoxicity Assay Kit (DoGen) following the manufacturer's protocol. Absorbances were read at 490 nm in the microplate reader.

2.4. Cell Death Assay

Cell death was measured by PI labeling. Cultured cells were stained with PI solution (2 μg/mL) in the dark at 37 °C for 30 min, observed under an inverted fluorescence microscope (Olympus IX73, Olympus, Tokyo, Japan) at 200× magnification, and the images were recorded.

2.5. Measurement of Intracellular ROS Levels

The DCFH-DA fluorescent dye probe was used to measure intracellular ROS production. After different treatments, cells were washed with PBS and incubated with 10 μM DCFH-DA in PBS at 37 °C for 20 min in the dark. The cells were washed twice with PBS, and fluorescent images were taken under a microscope at 200× magnification.

2.6. Extraction of Nuclear Protein

NF-κB p65 activity in the nuclear fractions was determined using a cell fractionation kit (Cell Signaling Technology) according to the manufacturer's instructions. The detailed procedure has been explained previously [24]. Briefly, after a treatment, cells were washed twice with cold PBS and lysed with a cytosol extraction buffer. The supernatant was collected by centrifugation at a maximum speed for 5 min. Finally, the nuclear fraction was separated using a nuclear extraction buffer. The supernatant containing the nuclear protein extract was transferred to a fresh microcentrifuge tube and stored at −20 °C.

2.7. Western Blotting

Cells were washed twice with PBS and then lysed in a radioimmunoprecipitation assay lysis buffer (Elpis Biotech, Daejeon, Korea) containing protease inhibitor cocktail tablets (Roche Diagnostics, Mannheim, Germany); following this, they were centrifuged at 14,000× *g* for 15 min. Protein concentration was measured using the bicinchoninic acid kit (BCA Protein Assay Kit; Pierce, Rockford, IL, USA). A standardized quantity (20 μg) of protein extract was electrophoresed, immunoblotted, and detected as reported previously [24].

2.8. Immunofluorescence Assay

Cultured cells were seeded onto a coverslip at a density of 2×10^5 cells/mL. After different treatments, the medium was discarded by draining, and the adhering cells were washed with PBS, fixed with 4% formaldehyde for 15 min, and permeabilized with 0.1% Triton X-100 for 10 min at room temperature. The cells were saturated with PBS containing 1% bovine serum albumin for 1 h at room temperature, then incubated with the relevant primary antibody (Cell Signaling Technology) at 1:100 dilution in PBS at 4 °C overnight. Next, cells were washed, stained with Alexa Fluor 488-conjugated goat anti-mouse antibodies (Invitrogen), and mounted with DAPI. The obtained images of the stained cells were measured quantitatively by ImageJ program (ImageJ software Version 1.54i, National Institute of Health, MD, USA).

2.9. Quantification of IL-1β and IL-18 via an Enzyme-Linked Immunosorbent Assay (ELISA)

The protein expression levels of IL-1β and IL-18 in the culture supernatant were measured using BD OptEIA ELISA kits (BD Biosciences, San Jose, CA, USA). Values were expressed as pg/mL based on standard curves of recombinant cytokines.

2.10. Statistical Analysis

GraphPad Prism 5 (GraphPad Software Prism 5 Version 5.03, Inc., La Jolla, CA, USA) was used to analyze all the data. The significance of differences between control and experimental values was assessed using the unpaired *t*-test or one-way analysis of variance. All values are expressed as mean ± standard error of the mean (SEM).

3. Results

3.1. Exposure to $PM_{2.5}$ Induced Cell Death in BEAS-2B Cells in a Dose-Dependent Manner

To explore the effect of $PM_{2.5}$ on cell death, BEAS-2B cell lines were treated with varying concentrations of $PM_{2.5}$ (0, 10, 20, and 40 μg/mL) for 24 h, in reference to previous studies [14,25]. As $PM_{2.5}$ directly affects in the airway and lungs, we selected the BEAS-2B cell lines, human bronchial epithelial cells. Cell viability in bronchial epithelial cells decreased significantly ($p < 0.05$) from a $PM_{2.5}$ concentration of 20 μg/mL, compared with the control group of no exposure to $PM_{2.5}$ (Figure 1A). As for cytotoxicity, Figure 1B shows that more LDH was released with an increasing concentration of $PM_{2.5}$. Cells with a PI signal, a surrogate marker of cell death, were more pronounced fluorescence uptake in a dose-dependent manner as determined by quantified fluorescence uptake (Figure 1C,D). Based on these results, 20 μg/mL of $PM_{2.5}$, which induced a marked inflammatory response with an acceptable cytotoxicity, was chosen for further experiments with various inhibitors.

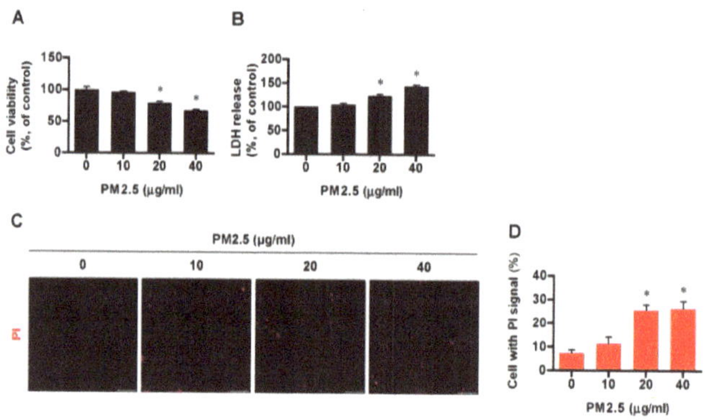

Figure 1. $PM_{2.5}$−induced cell death in BEAS−2B cells. Cells were treated with $PM_{2.5}$ at different concentrations (0, 10, 20, and 40 μg/mL) for 24 h. (**A**,**B**) Effects of $PM_{2.5}$ on the cell viability and the amount of LDH release in BEAS-2B cells. (**C**,**D**) Cell death assessed by PI uptake (red fluorescence) and the ratio of PI-positive cells using ImageJ software. All experiments were performed in triplicate. Values are the mean ± SEM. *, $p < 0.05$ compared with control; scale bar = 100 μm; LDH, lactate dehydrogenase; PI, propidium Iodide.

3.2. $PM_{2.5}$ Involved Activation of the NLRP3 Inflammasome and Release of IL-1β and IL-18 in BEAS-2B Cells

To determine whether the NLRP3 inflammasome is activated in BEAS-2B cells after $PM_{2.5}$ treatment, we measured the expression of NLRP3 inflammasome proteins, NLRP3, Casp1, and GSDMD-N. In Western blot analysis, the expression of NLRP3, Casp1, and GSMDM-N increased markedly with $PM_{2.5}$ treatment, especially at 20 and 40 μg/mL (Figure 2A–D). The levels of proinflammatory cytokines associated with pyroptosis, IL-1β, and IL-18 were significantly higher than in the control after $PM_{2.5}$ exposure (Figure 2E,F). In the immunofluorescence assay of NLRP3 and Casp1, the fluorescent intensity of the two vital mediators involved in pyroptosis became stronger as exposure to $PM_{2.5}$ increased (Figure 2G–J).

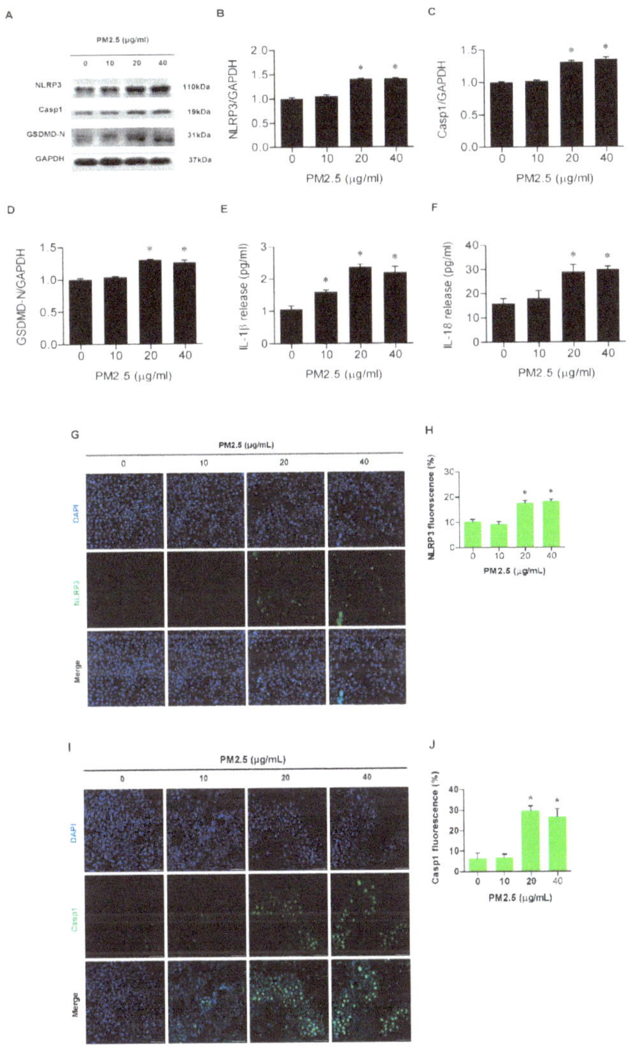

Figure 2. $PM_{2.5}$−induced activation of the NLRP3 inflammasome and release of IL−1β and IL−18 in BEAS−2B cells. Cells were treated with $PM_{2.5}$ at different concentrations (0, 10, 20, and 40 μg/mL) for 24 h. (**A–D**) Protein levels and densitometric analyses of NLRP3, Casp1, and GSDMD-N in cells. (**E,F**) Concentrations of IL−1β and IL−18 by ELISA. (**G,H**) NLRP3 detection by immunofluorescent staining and quantitation of the fluorescent signal. (**I,J**) Casp1 expression by immunofluorescent staining and quantification of its fluorescence intensity. All experiments were performed in triplicate. Values are the mean ± SEM. *, $p < 0.05$ compared with the control; scale bar = 100 μm.

3.3. $PM_{2.5}$ Exposure Triggered Pyroptosis in BEAS-2B Cells in a NLRP3-Inflammasome-Dependent Manner

To further confirm an effect of the NLRP3 inflammasome on pyroptosis induced by $PM_{2.5}$ in airway epithelial cells, BEAS-2B cells were treated for 2 h with MCC950, an NLRP3 inflammasome inhibitor, followed by a 24 h exposure to $PM_{2.5}$ of 20 μg/mL. The expressions of pyrotosis parameters such as NLRP3, Casp1, and GSDMD-N were significantly reduced by prior MCC950 administration with $PM_{2.5}$ exposure, compared to the $PM_{2.5}$-treated control

(Figure 3A–D). Moreover, LDH release and cells with positive PI staining decreased with MCC950 treatment and subsequent $PM_{2.5}$ exposure (Figure 3E–G). MCC950 also diminished the concentration of IL-1β and IL-18 (Figure 3H,I). Taken together, these results confirm that $PM_{2.5}$-induced pyroptosis in BEAS-2B cells is NLRP3-inflammasome-dependent.

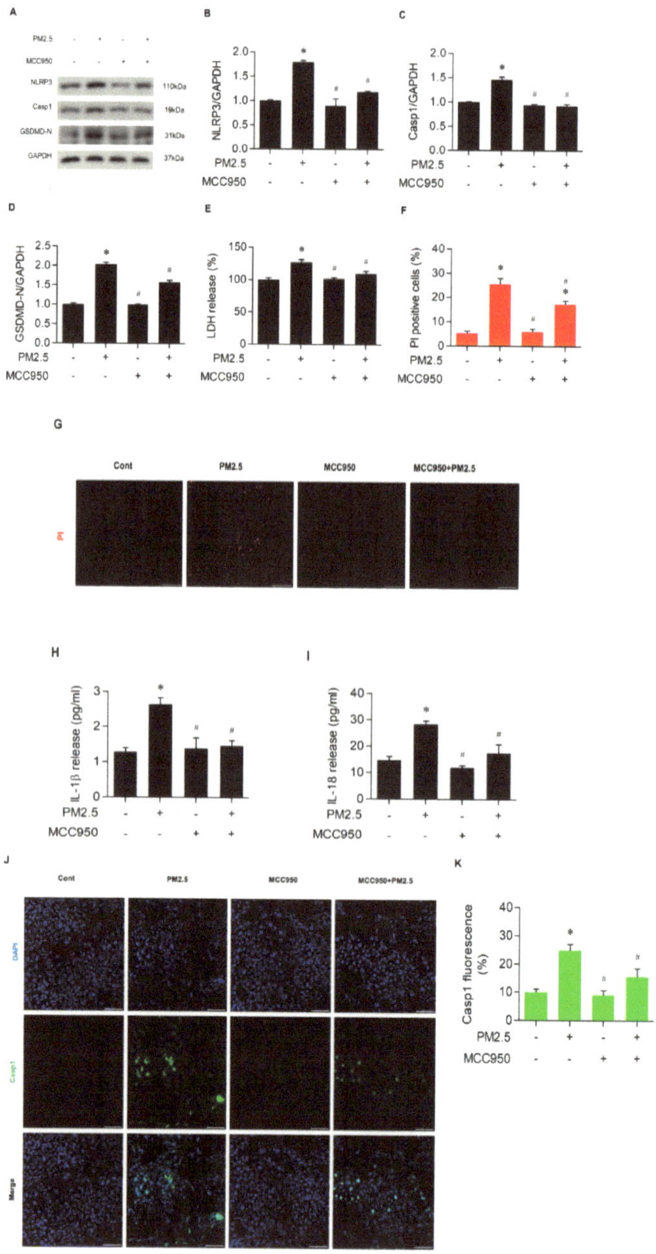

Figure 3. $PM_{2.5}$ triggered pyroptosis of BEAS−2B cells in an NLRP3−inflammasome−dependent manner. Cells were treated with $PM_{2.5}$ of 20 μg/mL for 24 h after treatment with MCC950, a NLRP3

inflammasome inhibitor (0.5 μM) for 2 h. (**A–D**) Western blotting results and quantitation analysis for NLRP3, Casp1, and GSDMD−N expression in BEAS−2B cells treated with MCC950 and exposed to $PM_{2.5}$ or not. (**E**) Effects of MCC950 on the amount of LDH release in $PM_{2.5}$-treated cells. (**F,G**) Effects of MCC950 on $PM_{2.5}$-induced PI staining in BEAS-2B cells. (**H,I**) Effect of MCC950 on IL−1β and IL−18 production in $PM_{2.5}$-treated cells. (**J,K**) Effect of MCC950 on Casp1 expression measured by immunofluorescent staining and quantification of its fluorescence intensity. All experiments were performed in triplicate. Values are the mean ± SEM. *, $p < 0.05$ compared with the control; #, $p < 0.05$ compared with the $PM_{2.5}$−treated control; scale bar = 100 μm. LDH, lactate dehydrogenase; PI, propidium Iodide.

3.4. *$PM_{2.5}$ Activated the ROS/NF-κB Pathway in BEAS-2B Cells*

Consistent with results of our previous studies [14,18], $PM_{2.5}$ at 20 μg/mL markedly increased intracellular ROS production in bronchial epithelial cells. However, prior treatment with 5 mM NAC, a ROS scavenger, for 1 h before the exposure to $PM_{2.5}$ significantly decreased the ROS level in cells compared with the NAC-untreated and $PM_{2.5}$-exposed control ($p < 0.05$) in the DCFH-DA fluorescence assay (Figure 4A,B). To investigate whether the increased ROS level participates in the activation of NF-κB in $PM_{2.5}$-treated cells, the expression of NF-κB p65 protein in cells treated with both NAC and $PM_{2.5}$ was examined by Western blotting. As shown in Figure 4C–E, $PM_{2.5}$ induced nuclear NF-κB p65 expression and increased fluorescence, but the effect was reversed by NAC administration. Therefore, we conclude that $PM_{2.5}$ activates the NF-κB signaling pathway by increasing the intracellular ROS level in BEAS-2B cells.

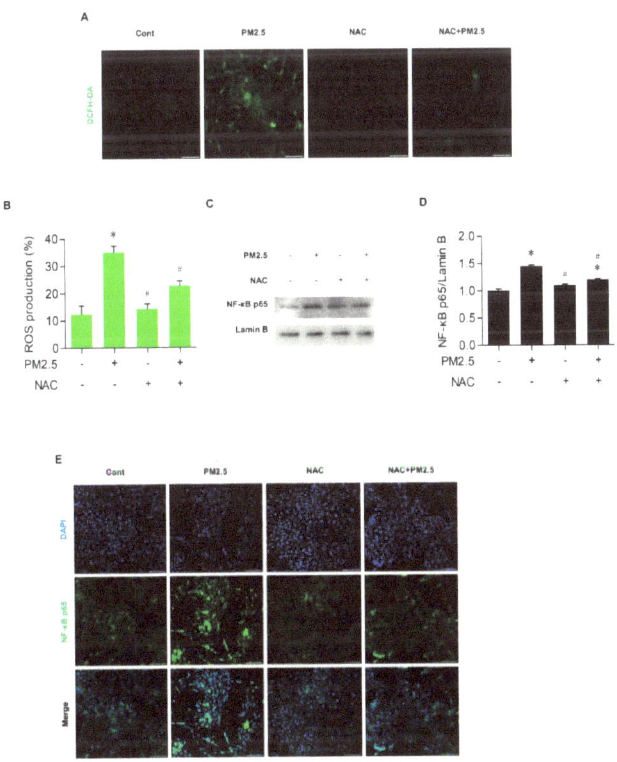

Figure 4. $PM_{2.5}$ activated the ROS/NF−κB pathway in BEAS−2B cells. Cells were treated with 5 mM NAC, a ROS scavenger, for 1 h, and then were treated with 20 μg/mL $PM_{2.5}$ for 24 h. (**A**) The intracellular

ROS levels shown by DCFH-DA fluorescence. (**B**) Relative intensity of ROS production in DCFH−DA fluorescence. (**C**) Expression of NF-κB p65 and lamin−B1 by Western blotting. (**D**) Quantitation of the relative density of NF-κB p65 to lamin−B1. (**E**) Nuclear localization of NF−κB p65 by immunofluorescence staining. All experiments were performed in triplicate. Values are the mean ± SEM. *, $p < 0.05$ compared with the control; #, $p < 0.05$ compared with the $PM_{2.5}$-treated control; scale bar = 50 μm.

3.5. *NAC Inhibited the Expression of NLRP3 and Casp1 in $PM_{2.5}$-Treated BEAS-2B Cells*

We evaluated whether increased ROS by $PM_{2.5}$ is associated with the activation of the NLRP3 inflammasome. Figure 5A–D shows that pretreatment with NAC before $PM_{2.5}$ exposure markedly decreased the level of NLRP3, Casp1, and GSDMD-N in BEAS-2B cells ($p < 0.05$). In the immunofluorescence method, the expression of NLRP3 was reduced significantly by NAC in $PM_{2.5}$-treated cells (Figure 5E,F). In addition, the change of Casp1 expression showed a similar pattern (Figure 5G,H). These findings support the notion that increased ROS generated by $PM_{2.5}$ is important for inducing NLRP3-inflammasome-mediated pyroptosis.

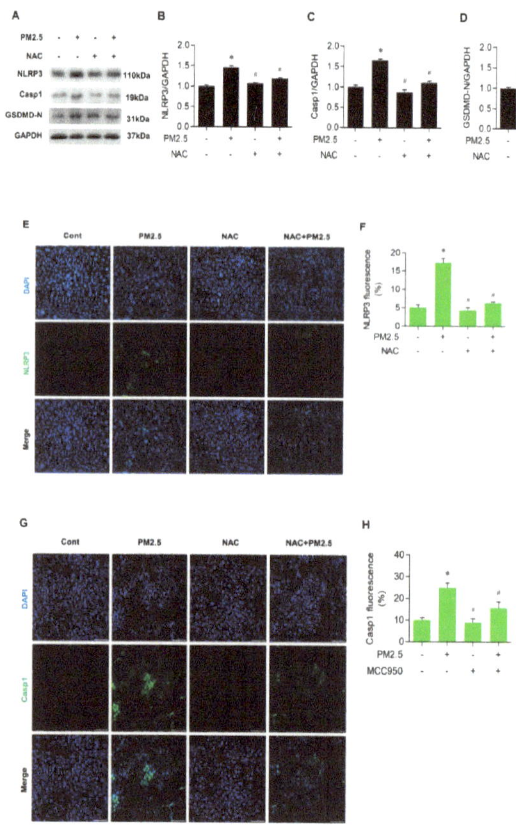

Figure 5. NAC inhibited the expression of NLRP3 and Casp1 in $PM_{2.5}$−treated BEAS−2B cells. Cells were treated with 5 mM NAC for 1 h and then administered with 20 μg/mL $PM_{2.5}$ for 24 h. (**A–D**) Protein levels and densitometric analyses of NLRP3, Casp1, and GSDMD−N in cells. (**E,F**) NLRP3 measured by immunofluorescent staining and quantified by the fluorescent signal. (**G,H**) Casp1 detection by immunofluorescent staining and its quantitation of the fluorescence intensity. All experiments were performed in triplicate. Values are the mean ± SEM. *, $p < 0.05$ compared with the control; #, $p < 0.05$ compared with the $PM_{2.5}$-treated control; scale bar = 100 μm.

3.6. BAY Diminished Pyroptotic Cell Death in $PM_{2.5}$-Treated BEAS-2B Cells

To further clarify the involvement of NF-κB signaling in the effect of ROS on pyroptosis caused by $PM_{2.5}$ exposure, cells were treated 10 μM BAY, an NF-κB inhibitor, for 30 min before exposure to $PM_{2.5}$ at 20 μg/mL for 24 h. As shown in Figure 6A, the cytotoxicity as measured by LDH level decreased significantly in cells previously treated with BAY compared with activity in cells exposed to $PM_{2.5}$ only. In addition, BAY significantly decreased the proportion of PI-positive cells caused by $PM_{2.5}$ exposure (Figure 6B,C). The expression of NLRP3 and Casp1, the crucial players in pyroptosis, were lowered considerably by BAY treatment in the immunofluorescence assay with $PM_{2.5}$ exposure (Figure 6D,G). Collectively, these results provide strong evidence that the activation of NF-κB signaling pathway is involved in $PM_{2.5}$-induced cell pyroptosis in BEAS-2B cells.

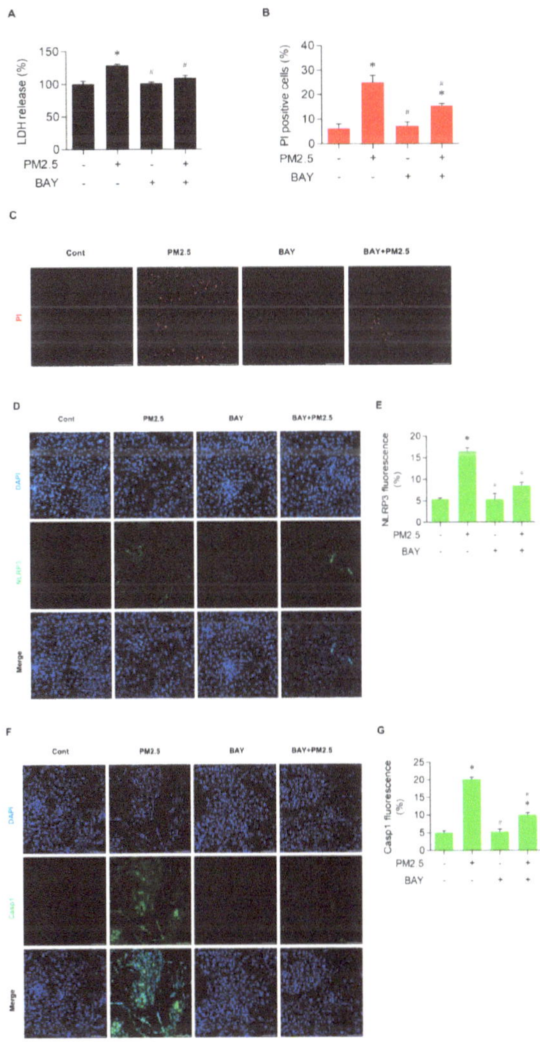

Figure 6. BAY, a NF−κB inhibitor, alleviated pyroptotic cell death in $PM_{2.5}$−treated BEAS−2B cells. Cells were treated with 10 μM BAY for 30 min, followed by 20 μg/mL $PM_{2.5}$ for 24 h. (**A**) Cytotoxicity as measured by the amount of LDH release. (**B**,**C**) PI−stained cell death with the ratio of PI−positive

cells quantified by ImageJ software. (**D**,**E**) Effect of BAY on NLRP3 expression detected in immunofluorescence and the quantification of its fluorescence. (**F**,**G**) Effect of BAY on Casp1 measured by immunofluorescent staining and its fluorescent intensity. For all experiments, triplicated data are shown as mean ± SEM. *, $p < 0.05$ compared with the control; #, $p < 0.05$ compared with the $PM_{2.5}$-treated control; scale bar = 100 μm.

4. Discussion

In this study, we demonstrated that $PM_{2.5}$ exposure induces pyroptosis and production of the proinflammatory cytokines IL-1β and IL-18 via the NLRP3 inflammasome in bronchial epithelial cells and that the effect is modulated by activating the ROS/NF-κB signaling pathway.

$PM_{2.5}$ causes cytotoxicities by regulating ROS-induced cell death pathways such as apoptosis, autophagy, and pyroptosis. Newly discovered cell death pathways such as ferropotosis by iron-dependent lipid peroxidation and necroptosis, a form of caspase-independent programmed necrosis, could also be affected by $PM_{2.5}$ via ROS stimuli [26]. Various factors such as differences in dose or duration of $PM_{2.5}$ exposure, the nature of components in $PM_{2.5}$, and the types of cells or organs involved could affect the specific profile of cell death pathways. As for pyroptosis, the best-known involved process is a classical or canonical inflammasome-induced pathway mediated by Casp1 and executed by GSDMD [27]. We also verified that $PM_{2.5}$ exposure causes pyroptotic cell death in a dose-dependent manner by ROS generation through the NLRP3-inflammasome-induced classical pathway as shown by our step-by-step experiments with the ROS scavenger NAC and the NLRP3 inhibitor MCC950.

The airway epithelium is a primary line of defense against exogenous insults in the respiratory tract. It plays a critical role as a physical barrier as well as in inflammation and innate immune responses. Previous in vitro research on pyroptosis in $PM_{2.5}$ exposure has focused on alveolar macrophages, the main inflammatory cells in the lung [28,29]. There have been few studies of the effect of $PM_{2.5}$ on pyroptosis in airway epithelial cells. In the present study, we have confirmed that the ROS–NLRP3 inflammasome–Casp1–GSDMD axis is activated in bronchial epithelial cells exposed to $PM_{2.5}$. Based on the fact that defects in the airway epithelium are closely associated with asthma, COPD, cystic fibrosis, and infection [30], the bronchial epithelial cell injury caused by pyroptosis after PM exposure could have an impact on the pathogenesis of various respiratory diseases. Interestingly, Ren et al. reported that pathways other than pyroptosis, such as apoptosis or cell cycle arrest, occur via upregulating ROS after $PM_{2.5}$ exposure and lead to cell damage in a macrophage cell line [29]. Further research is needed to explore what the most dominant pathways in the various cytotoxicities are and how they interact with different $PM_{2.5}$ exposures.

This study determined that the NF-κB signaling pathway participates in pyroptotic cell death by ROS regulation in bronchial epithelial cells after $PM_{2.5}$ treatment; an experiment with NF-κB inhibitor showed reduced expression of Casp1, with decreased LDH concentrations and fewer PI positive cells. NF-κB is a key transcriptional factor with a critical role in inflammation and cell death pathways. Because an activated NF-κB signal induces NLRP3 inflammasome expression and production of proinflammatory cytokines such as IL-1β [31,32], it could trigger and maintain pyroptosis. Some evidence shows that ROS release by $PM_{2.5}$ exposure activates NF-κB signaling and enhances a downstream inflammatory cascade in airway epithelial cells [31,33]. Further, Song et al. demonstrated that regulation of mir-331 expression by $PM_{2.5}$ exposure with ROS generation maintains NF-κB signaling activation in human airway epithelium [31]. In addition, $PM_{2.5}$-induced apoptosis or autophagy also involve the NF-κB pathway [26]. Dou et al. reported that cooking-oil-fume-derived $PM_{2.5}$ activates the MAPK/NF-κB/STAT1 pathway and results in inflammation as well as apoptosis and cell damage [34]. IL-1β is one of the major proinflammatory cytokines, produced in a proactive form by some types of immune cells such as macrophages or dendritic cells. It exerts biologic effects after transformation to its active form and extracellular secretion through pyroptosis. It increases pulmonary inflammation and fibrosis by inducing neutrophil and macrophage infiltrations and disruption of elastic fiber in alveoli, with increased matrix metalloproteinases, MMP-9 and MMP-12 [35]. Additionally, IL-1β has a substantial role in lung cancer development via regulation of tumor growth, invasiveness, and angiogenesis, which were demonstrated in a clinical study using the anti-IL-1β antibody canakinumab [36]. Unlike IL-1β, IL-18 is produced in various cell types, but like IL-1β it is stored as a proactive form to be activated by Casp1 in the NLRP3 inflammasome. IL-18 has pleotropic functions depending on cell type and the cytokine milieu, such as production of interferon-γ (IFN-γ) as well as the other cytokines IL-4 and IL-13. In an animal model study by Sugimoto et al., IL-18 with antigen activated Th1 cells with the production of IFN-γ, IL-19, and IL-13, leading to severe asthma development [37]. We observed that IL-1β and IL-18 were released by $PM_{2.5}$ exposure in an NLRP3-inflammasome-dependent manner in bronchial epithelial cell lines, which could induce lung injury.

There are some weaknesses to be addressed in this work. We conducted an in vitro study using the bronchial epithelial cell line and did not verify in vitro experiments, which could limit the generalizability of our findings. In addition, we focused mainly on the ROS/NF-κB signal pathway in the $PM_{2.5}$-induced pyroptosis. A recent study showed that hexavalent chromium, one of the major components in $PM_{2.5}$, induces inflammasome-mediated pyroptosis in airway epithelial cells [38]. Further research on this topic is needed for a better understanding of $PM_{2.5}$-related toxicity and target development to reverse its harmful effects. Lastly, we chose the concentration of $PM_{2.5}$ based on the results of cell cytotoxicity and viability. However, the exposed level of $PM_{2.5}$ in this experimental setting might not be similar to it in a real-world situation. This could be another limitation in the interpretation of our findings. Various diseases such as multiple sclerosis, inflammatory bowel diseases, autoimmune thyroiditis, anti-synthetase syndrome, as well as myocardial infarction, are associated with NLRP3 inflammasome [39–41]. As we revealed that NLRP3 inflammasome is activated and induces pyroptotic cell injury via ROS/NF-κB signal by $PM_{2.5}$ exposure, targeting mediators involved in this cascade would be a potential therapeutic option for those intractable diseases.

In conclusion, this study has shown that $PM_{2.5}$ induces pyroptosis in airway epithelial cells via the ROS–NLRP3 inflammasome–Casp1–GSDMD axis with NF-κB signaling activation. Considering that pyroptosis might be involved in various respiratory diseases such as asthma, COPD, and lung cancer and that $PM_{2.5}$ is one of the most important factors in those diseases' pathogenesis, these findings provide valuable clues to explore new therapeutic candidates in pulmonary diseases aggravated by $PM_{2.5}$.

Author Contributions: J.-Y.K.: data curation, writing—original draft preparation, reviewing, and editing. D.-C.L.: conceptualization, investigation, supervision, reviewing, and editing. H.C.: data curation, formal analysis, methodology, visualization, reviewing, and editing. J.-M.O.: data curation, visualization, investigation. M.K.: investigation, methodology, reviewing, and editing. All authors have read and agreed to the published version of the manuscript.

Funding: This research was supported by the Clinical Research Institute grant (CMCDJ-P-2022-019) funded by The Catholic University of Korea Daejeon St. Mary's Hospital, as well as the 2022 Alumni Research Fund of the Catholic University of Korea College of Medicine Alumni Association. The funders had no role in the study design, data collection and analysis, decision to publish, or preparation of the manuscript.

Institutional Review Board Statement: The study protocol was approved by the Institutional Review Board of Daejeon St. Mary's Hospital (IRB No. CMCDJ-AP-2022-004).

Informed Consent Statement: Not available.

Data Availability Statement: Data will be available from the corresponding author on reasonable request.

Conflicts of Interest: The authors declare no conflicts of interest.

Abbreviations

BEGM: bronchial epithelial growth medium; Casp 1, caspase-1; COPD, chronic obstructive pulmonary disease; ELISA, enzyme-linked immunosorbent assay; GSDM, gasdermin; GSDMD-N, N-terminal gasdermin D; IL, interleukin; LDH, lactate dehydrogenase; NAC, N-acetylcysteine; NF-κB: nuclear factor-κB; NLRP3, NOD-like receptor protein-3; PI, propidium iodide; PM, particulate matter; ROS, reactive oxygen species.

References

1. Cui, A.; Xiang, M.; Xu, M.; Lu, P.; Wang, S.; Zou, Y.; Qiao, K.; Jin, C.; Li, Y.; Lu, M.; et al. VCAM-1-mediated neutrophil infiltration exacerbates ambient fine particle-induced lung injury. *Toxicol. Lett.* **2019**, *302*, 60–74. [CrossRef]
2. Health Effects Institute. *State of Global Air 2020*; Health Effects Institute: Boston, MA, USA, 2020.
3. Trasande, L.; Malecha, P.; Attina, T.M. Particulate Matter Exposure and Preterm Birth: Estimates of U.S. Attributable Burden and Economic Costs. *Environ. Health Perspect.* **2016**, *124*, 1913–1918. [CrossRef]
4. Cohen, A.J.; Brauer, M.; Burnett, R.; Anderson, H.R.; Frostad, J.; Estep, K.; Balakrishnan, K.; Brunekreef, B.; Dandona, L.; Dandona, R.; et al. Estimates and 25-year trends of the global burden of disease attributable to ambient air pollution: An analysis of data from the Global Burden of Diseases Study. *Lancet* **2017**, *389*, 1907–1918. [CrossRef]
5. Li, C.Y.; Wu, C.D.; Pan, W.C.; Chen, Y.C.; Su, H.J. Association Between Long-term Exposure to $PM_{2.5}$ and Incidence of Type 2 Diabetes in Taiwan: A National Retrospective Cohort Study. *Epidemiology* **2019**, *30* (Suppl. S1), S67–S75. [CrossRef] [PubMed]
6. Coleman, N.C.; Burnett, R.T.; Ezzati, M.; Marshall, J.D.; Robinson, A.L.; Pope, C.A., 3rd. Fine Particulate Matter Exposure and Cancer Incidence: Analysis of SEER Cancer Registry Data from 1992–2016. *Environ. Health Perspect.* **2020**, *128*, 107004. [CrossRef] [PubMed]
7. Yang, X.; Zhang, T.; Zhang, Y.; Chen, H.; Sang, S. Global burden of COPD attributable to ambient $PM_{2.5}$ in 204 countries and territories, 1990 to 2019: A systematic analysis for the Global Burden of Disease Study. *Sci. Total. Environ.* **2019**, *796*, 148819. [CrossRef]
8. GBD 2019 Risk Factors Collaborators. Global burden of 87 risk factors in 204 countries and territories, 1990–2019: A systematic analysis for the Global Burden of Disease Study. *Lancet* **2019**, *396*, 1223–1249. [CrossRef]
9. Sang, S.; Chu, C.; Zhang, T.; Chen, H.; Yang, X. The global burden of disease attributable to ambient fine particulate matter in 204 countries and territories, 1990–2019: A systematic analysis of the Global Burden of Disease Study 2019. *Ecotoxicol. Environ. Saf.* **2022**, *238*, 113588. [CrossRef]
10. Risom, L.; Møller, P.; Loft, S. Oxidative stress-induced DNA damage by particulate air pollution. *Mutat. Res.* **2005**, *592*, 119–137. [CrossRef]
11. Abbas, I.; Badran, G.; Verdin, A.; Ledoux, F.; Roumie, M.; Lo Guidice, J.M.; Courcot, D.; Garçon, G. In vitro evaluation of organic extractable matter from ambient $PM_{2.5}$ using human bronchial epithelial BEAS-2B cells: Cytotoxicity, oxidative stress, pro-inflammatory response, genotoxicity, and cell cycle deregulation. *Environ. Res.* **2019**, *171*, 510–522. [CrossRef]
12. Sachdeva, K.; Do, D.C.; Zhang, Y.; Hu, X.; Chen, J.; Gao, P. Environmental Exposures and Asthma Development: Autophagy, Mitophagy, and Cellular Senescence. *Front. Immunol.* **2019**, *10*, 2787. [CrossRef]
13. Kim, J.S.; Choi, H.; Oh, J.M.; Kim, Y.H.; Kim, S.W.; Kim, S.W.; Kim, B.G.; Cho, J.H.; Lee, J.; Lee, D.C. Effect of fluticasone propionate on human nasal fibroblasts exposed to urban particulate matter. *Auris Nasus Larynx* **2020**, *47*, 415–424. [CrossRef]
14. Lee, D.C.; Oh, J.M.; Choi, H.; Kim, S.W.; Kim, S.W.; Kim, B.G.; Cho, J.H.; Lee, J.; Kim, J.-S. Eupatilin Inhibits Reactive Oxygen Species Generation via Akt/NF-κB/MAPK Signaling Pathways in Particulate Matter-Exposed Human Bronchial Epithelial Cells. *Toxics* **2021**, *9*, 38. [CrossRef]
15. Gonzalez-Gonzalez, F.J.; Chandel, N.S.; Jain, M.; Budinger, G.R.S. Reactive oxygen species as signaling molecules in the development of lung fibrosis. *Transl. Res.* **2017**, *190*, 61–68. [CrossRef] [PubMed]
16. Boukhenouna, S.; Wilson, M.A.; Bahmed, K.; Kosmider, B. Reactive Oxygen Species in Chronic Obstructive Pulmonary Disease. *Oxid. Med. Cell. Longev.* **2018**, *2018*, 5730395. [CrossRef] [PubMed]
17. Yang, L.; Li, C.; Tang, X. The Impact of $PM_{2.5}$ on the Host Defense of Respiratory System. *Front. Cell Dev. Biol.* **2020**, *8*, 91. [CrossRef] [PubMed]
18. Lee, D.C.; Choi, H.; Oh, J.M.; Lee, J.; Lee, J.; Lee, H.Y.; Kang, J.Y. Urban particulate matter regulates tight junction proteins by inducing oxidative stress via the Akt signal pathway in human nasal epithelial cells. *Toxicol. Lett.* **2020**, *333*, 33–41. [CrossRef] [PubMed]
19. Shi, J.; Gao, W.; Shao, F. Pyroptosis: Gasdermin-Mediated Programmed Necrotic Cell Death. *Trends Biochem. Sci.* **2017**, *42*, 245–254. [CrossRef]
20. Feng, Y.; Li, M.; Yangzhong, X.; Zhang, X.; Zu, A.; Hou, Y.; Li, L.; Sun, S. Pyroptosis in inflammation-related respiratory disease. *J. Physiol. Biochem.* **2022**, *78*, 721–737. [CrossRef]
21. Tsai, Y.M.; Chiang, K.H.; Hung, J.Y.; Chang, W.A.; Lin, H.P.; Shieh, J.M.; Chong, I.; Hsu, Y. Der f1 induces pyroptosis in human bronchial epithelia via the NLRP3 inflammasome. *Int. J. Mol. Med.* **2018**, *41*, 757–764. [CrossRef]

22. Liu, T.; Zhou, Y.T.; Wang, L.Q.; Li, L.Y.; Bao, Q.; Tian, S.; Chen, M.X.; Chen, H.X.; Cui, J.; Li, C.W. NOD-like receptor family, pyrin domain containing 3 (NLRP3) contributes to inflammation, pyroptosis, and mucin production in human airway epithelium on rhinovirus infection. *J. Allergy Clin. Immunol.* **2019**, *144*, 777–787.e9. [CrossRef] [PubMed]
23. Zhang, M.Y.; Jiang, Y.X.; Yang, Y.C.; Liu, J.Y.; Huo, C.; Ji, X.L.; Qu, Y.-Q. Cigarette smoke extract induces pyroptosis in human bronchial epithelial cells through the ROS/NLRP3/caspase-1 pathway. *Life Sci.* **2021**, *269*, 119090. [CrossRef]
24. Lee, D.C.; Choi, H.; Oh, J.M.; Hong, Y.; Jeong, S.H.; Kim, C.S.; Kim, D.-K.; Cho, W.-K.; Kim, S.W.; Kim, S.W.; et al. The effect of urban particulate matter on cultured human nasal fibroblasts. *Int. Forum Allergy Rhinol.* **2018**, *8*, 993–1000. [CrossRef] [PubMed]
25. Bang, J.; Son, K.H.; Heo, H.-R.; Park, E.; Kwak, H.-J.; Uhm, K.-O.; Chung, M.-H.; Kim, Y.-Y.; Lim, H.J. Exogenous 8-Hydroxydeoxyguanosine Attenuates $PM_{2.5}$-Induced Inflammation in Human Bronchial Epithelial Cells by Decreasing NLRP3 Inflammasome Activation. *Antioxidants* **2023**, *12*, 1189. [CrossRef] [PubMed]
26. Chen, Y.; Wu, Y.; Qi, Y.; Liu, S. Cell Death Pathways: The Variable Mechanisms Underlying Fine Particulate Matter-Induced Cytotoxicity. *ACS Nanosci. Au* **2023**, *3*, 130–139. [CrossRef] [PubMed]
27. Wu, Y.; Zhang, J.; Yu, S.; Li, Y.; Zhu, J.; Zhang, K.; Zhang, R. Cell pyroptosis in health and inflammatory diseases. *Cell Death Discov.* **2022**, *8*, 191. [CrossRef] [PubMed]
28. Li, J.; An, Z.; Song, J.; Du, J.; Zhang, L.; Jiang, J.; Ma, Y.; Wang, C.; Zhang, J.; Wu, W. Fine particulate matter-induced lung inflammation is mediated by pyroptosis in mice. *Ecotoxicol. Environ. Saf.* **2021**, *219*, 112351. [CrossRef]
29. Ren, F.; Xu, J.; Zhang, J.; Xu, X.; Huang, L.; Sun, W.; Li, R.; Li, F. $PM_{2.5}$ induced lung injury through upregulating ROS-dependent NLRP3 Inflammasome-Mediated Pyroptosis. *Immunobiology* **2022**, *227*, 152207. [CrossRef]
30. Hiemstra, P.S.; McCray, P.B., Jr.; Bals, R. The innate immune function of airway epithelial cells in inflammatory lung disease. *Eur. Respir. J.* **2015**, *45*, 1150–1162. [CrossRef]
31. Nam, H.Y.; Choi, B.H.; Lee, J.Y.; Lee, S.G.; Kim, Y.H.; Lee, K.H.; Yoon, H.K.; Song, J.S.; Kim, H.J.; Lim, Y. The role of nitric oxide in the particulate matter ($PM_{2.5}$)-induced NFkappaB activation in lung epithelial cells. *Toxicol. Lett.* **2004**, *148*, 95–102. [CrossRef]
32. Guo, H.; Callaway, J.B.; Ting, J.P. Inflammasomes: Mechanism of action, role in disease, and therapeutics. *Nat. Med.* **2015**, *21*, 677–687. [CrossRef] [PubMed]
33. Song, L.; Li, D.; Li, X.; Ma, L.; Bai, X.; Wen, Z.; Zhang, X.; Chen, D.; Peng, L. Exposure to $PM_{2.5}$ induces aberrant activation of NF-κB in human airway epithelial cells by downregulating miR-331 expression. *Environ. Toxicol. Pharmacol.* **2017**, *50*, 192–199. [CrossRef]
34. Dou, C.; Zhang, J.; Qi, C. Cooking oil fume-derived $PM_{2.5}$ induces apoptosis in A549 cells and MAPK/NF-κB/STAT1 pathway activation. *Environ. Sci. Pollut. Res.* **2018**, *25*, 9940–9948. [CrossRef] [PubMed]
35. Lappalainen, U.; Whitsett, J.A.; Wert, S.E.; Tichelaar, J.W.; Bry, K. Interleukin-1beta causes pulmonary inflammation, emphysema, and airway remodeling in the adult murine lung. *Am. J. Respir. Cell Mol. Biol.* **2005**, *32*, 311–318. [CrossRef] [PubMed]
36. Ridker, P.M.; MacFadyen, J.G.; Thuren, T.; Everett, B.M.; Libby, P.; Glynn, R.J. Effect of interleukin-1β inhibition with canakinumab on incident lung cancer in patients with atherosclerosis: Exploratory results from a randomised, double-blind, placebo-controlled trial. *Lancet* **2017**, *390*, 1833–1842. [CrossRef] [PubMed]
37. Sugimoto, T.; Ishikawa, Y.; Yoshimoto, T.; Hayashi, N.; Fujimoto, J.; Nakanishi, K. Interleukin 18 acts on memory T helper cells type 1 to induce airway inflammation and hyperresponsiveness in a naive host mouse. *J. Exp. Med.* **2004**, *199*, 535–545. [CrossRef]
38. Moonwiriyakit, A.; Dinsuwannakol, S.; Sontikun, J.; Timpratueang, K.; Muanprasat, C.; Khemawoot, P. Fine particulate matter $PM_{2.5}$ and its constituent, hexavalent chromium induce acute cytotoxicity in human airway epithelial cells via inflammasome-mediated pyroptosis. *Environ. Toxicol. Pharmacol.* **2024**, *107*, 104416. [CrossRef]
39. Ramos-Martinez, E.; Vega-Sánchez, A.E.; Pérez-Rubio, G.; Mejia, M.; Buendía-Roldán, I.; González-Pérez, M.I.; Mateos-Toledo, H.N.; Andrade, W.A.; Falfán-Valencia, R.; Rojas-Serrano, J. Enhanced Activity of NLRP3 Inflammasome in the Lung of Patients with Anti-Synthetase Syndrome. *Cells* **2020**, *12*, 60. [CrossRef]
40. Guo, Q.; Wu, Y.; Hou, Y.; Liu, Y.; Liu, T.; Zhang, H.; Fan, C.; Guan, H.; Li, Y.; Shan, Z.; et al. Cytokine Secretion and Pyroptosis of Thyroid Follicular Cells Mediated by Enhanced NLRP3, NLRP1, NLRC4, and AIM2 Inflammasomes Are Associated With Autoimmune Thyroiditis. *Front. Immunol.* **2018**, *9*, 1197. [CrossRef]
41. Fusco, R.; Siracusa, R.; Genovese, T.; Cuzzocrea, S.; Di Paola, R. Focus on the Role of NLRP3 Inflammasome in Diseases. *Int. J. Mol. Sci.* **2020**, *21*, 4223. [CrossRef]

medicina

MDPI

Systematic Review

Optimal Timing and Treatment Modalities of Arytenoid Dislocation and Subluxation: A Meta-Analysis

Andrea Frosolini [1,*,†], Valeria Caragli [2,†], Giulio Badin [3], Leonardo Franz [4], Patrizia Bartolotta [5], Andrea Lovato [6], Luca Vedovelli [5], Elisabetta Genovese [2], Cosimo de Filippis [4] and Gino Marioni [4]

1 Maxillofacial Surgery Unit, Department of Medical Biotechnologies, University of Siena, 53100 Siena, Italy
2 Otorhinolaryngology-Head and Neck Surgery, Audiology Program, Department of Diagnostic Clinical and Public Health, University of Modena and Reggio Emilia, 41125 Modena, Italy; valeria.caragli@unimore.it (V.C.); elisabetta.genovese@unimore.it (E.G.)
3 Otolaryngology Section, Department of Neuroscience DNS, University of Padova, 35100 Padova, Italy; badingiulio@gmail.com
4 Phoniatrics and Audiology Unit, Department of Neuroscience DNS, University of Padova, 31100 Treviso, Italy; leonardo.franz@unipd.it (L.F.); cosimo.defilippis@unipd.it (C.d.F.); gino.marioni@unipd.it (G.M.)
5 Unit of Biostatistics, Epidemiology, and Public Health, Department of Cardiac, Thoracic, Vascular Sciences, and Public Health, University of Padova, 35100 Padova, Italy; patrizia.bartolotta@ubep.unipd.it (P.B.); luca.vedovelli@ubep.unipd.it (L.V.)
6 Otorhinolaryngology Unit, Department of Surgical Specialties, Vicenza Civil Hospital, 36100 Vicenza, Italy; andrea.lovato.3@hotmail.it
* Correspondence: andreafrosolini@gmail.com
† These authors contributed equally to this work.

Abstract: *Background and Objective*: Arytenoid dislocation (AD) and subluxation (AS) impact vocal fold mobility, potentially affecting the quality of life. Their management, including the timing and modality of treatment, remains a subject of research. Our primary objective was to assess and compare the available treatment strategies for AS and AD. *Material and methods*: the protocol was registered on PROSPERO (CRD42023407521). Manuscripts retrieved from a previously published systematic review were evaluated. To comprehensively cover the last 25 years, an updated literature search was conducted, screening PubMed, Scopus, and Cochrane databases. Review Methods: We included studies that reported treatment modalities and the time to treatment (TT) for AS/AD, with outcomes objectively evaluated. Data on treatment success were pooled, and the impact of TT on recovery outcomes was analyzed. *Results*: Thirteen studies involving 361 patients were included. The majority of cases were attributed to iatrogenic trauma following intubation. Closed reduction (CR) was the primary treatment, with high success rates for both general (success rate: 77%, CI: 62–87%) and local anesthesia (success rate: 89%, CI: 70–97%). The standardized mean difference for the TT effect on treatment outcome was −1.24 (CI: −2.20 to −0.29). *Conclusions*: The absence of randomized controlled trials and the overall moderate-to-low quality of the studies highlighted the importance of the finding's careful interpretation. This meta-analysis underscores the effectiveness of CR in managing AS/AD, with both general and local anesthesia yielding high success rates. The findings highlight the importance of TT, suggesting that early intervention is paramount. Future clinical research is needed to further refine these findings and optimize treatment protocols.

Keywords: arytenoid dislocation; arytenoid subluxation; treatment; local anesthesia; general anesthesia; time to treatment

1. Introduction

The cricoarytenoid joint is included within a complex muscular and ligament system, and it is characterized by an elaborate three-dimensional movement pattern, the biomechanics of which have been effectively studied through 3D modelling and vector analysis [1,2]. The cricoarytenoid joint takes on a central role in the laryngeal function as it regulates the position, tension and volume of the vocal cords, allowing the protection of the airways, cough, ventilation control, and phonation [1]. Anatomically, it is a diarthrodial joint, supported by a wide joint capsule and strengthened posteriorly by the cricoarytenoid ligament [3].

Arytenoid dislocation (AD) and subluxation (AS) are defined as a complete or partial loss of contact between the cartilaginous surfaces, respectively [4]. It is an uncommon pathological condition with iatrogenic trauma due to intubation being the most frequent etiology (the reported percentage of AS/AD due to intubation ranges from 77.8% to 87.6%), followed by external blunt trauma (12.4% to 15.9% of cases) while spontaneous AS/AD is rare [5]. More precise estimates of the incidence of arytenoid dislocation following endotracheal intubation have been recently provided, reporting a pooled incidence rate of 0.093% (95% CI: 0.045–0.14%) according to a meta-analysis [6]. However, the reported incidence varies significantly across studies, likely due to differences in the population studied, diagnostic criteria, and underdiagnosis in clinical practice. The identified risk factors include anemia, laryngomalacia, acromegaly, chronic steroid use, low BMI, and conditions such as Marfan syndrome, renal failure, GERD, and CHARGE syndrome [5]. Moreover, procedural factors during anesthesia and surgery may increase AS/AD risk: cardiovascular surgery has been associated with an incidence of 0.07%, which is potentially linked to transesophageal echocardiography, while bariatric surgery involving a calibrating oro-gastric tube showed a postoperative incidence of 0.8% [6]. The presence of debilitating symptoms, including hoarseness, dysphonia, dysphagia, and dyspnoea, requires the active collaboration of the patient and a need for specific diagnostic tools and specialist consultation (i.e., an otolaryngologist or a phoniatrician) [7]. As mentioned above, given that the most frequent etiology is iatrogenic following intubation [5], in some cases, the diagnosis could be delayed due to difficulty in communicating with the patient during intensive care unit hospitalization [7]. Although cases of spontaneous resolution have been documented, this clinical situation usually requires adequate and timely treatment, as it could lead to a hypermobile joint or ankylosis resulting from hemarthrosis [8,9]. The most widely used treatment of AS/AD is closed reduction (CR) under general anesthesia. More recently, CR under local anesthesia, first described in 1978, has also become established [10]. Both techniques have shown good success rates [5], albeit local anesthesia techniques more frequently need to be repeated to achieve reduction than the technique under general anesthesia [11]. A single-centre retrospective study conducted on 35 patients concluded that the appropriate time window to perform CR under local anesthesia was between the 13th and 26th day after arytenoid dislocation [12]. It was assumed that premature treatment might not be effective because inflammation, pain, mucosal swelling, and hematoma in the early period of injury could hamper the surgical technique, while delayed treatment could be limited by cartilage fibrosis and joint stiffness [12]. In the largest series reported in the literature about AS/AD, accounting for 63 patients treated in a single institution with CR under general anesthesia, patients with complete voice improvement received earlier treatment (average of 14.3 weeks), while those with significant and slight improvement had longer times to treatment (averages of 97.2 weeks and 279.9 weeks, respectively).

Recently, our group undertook an in-depth examination of the literature related to the prevalence, symptoms, and diagnosis of AS/AD. Nevertheless, we did not focus on a detailed qualitative and quantitative analysis of the available treatment methods [5]. The main purpose of the present updated systematic review and meta-analysis was to provide a comprehensive overview of the current treatment options for AS and AD, highlighting the most effective treatment for managing this uncommon condition. A secondary aim was to investigate the importance of time to treatment (TT) in influencing AS and AD outcomes and prognoses.

2. Materials and Methods

2.1. Protocol Registration and Research Question

The protocol for the present systematic review and meta-analysis was registered on PROSPERO (study ID CRD42023407521) in February 2023, and it is available in its full version at https://www.crd.york.ac.uk/prospero/ (accessed on 5 January 2025).

The research question of the present review was twofold: Is the recently proposed closed reduction under local anesthesia significantly more effective for treating AS/AD compared to closed reduction under general anesthesia? Additionally, is the interval between the diagnosis and treatment a valid prognostic factor? Therefore, according to the Population, Intervention, Comparison, Outcomes (PICO) criteria, this study focused on the following: (i) a population of patients with a clinically confirmed diagnosis of AS/AD; (ii) the intervention of closed reduction; (iii) a comparison if reported, but not mandatory; and (iv) outcomes defined as the successful relocation of the arytenoid—observed via video laryngoscopy—tacking into account TT as a prognostic factor.

2.2. Eligibility Criteria

Studies were included when the following general criteria were met: (i) original articles including clinically confirmed cases of AS or AD with detailed information about its diagnostic workout; (ii) the availability of information about the treatment modality and TT; and (iii) defined outcomes in terms of AS or AD reduction confirmed by video laryngoscopy and/or computerized tomography. Exclusion criteria were as follows: (i) study design in the form of a case report, editorial, letter to the editor, or review; (ii) a non-English language study.

2.3. Information Sources—Electronic Database Search

Electronic databases were searched for papers about AS/AD over the last 25 years. The first part of the research (from 1 December 1999 to 1 December 2019) was covered in the previous publication [5], while updated research regarded papers published from 1 December 2019 to 1 August 2024 on PubMed, Scopus and Cochrane. The search terms were "arytenoid dislocation" and "arytenoid subluxation", separated by the Boolean operator "OR". The "Related articles" option on the PubMed homepage was also considered. Titles and abstracts of papers available in the English language were examined by three authors (V.C., B.G., and A.F.). The identified full texts were screened for original data, and the related references were retrieved and checked manually for other relevant studies.

2.4. Data Extraction and Qualitative Assessment

Three authors (V.C., B.G., and A.F.) performed the data extraction and qualitative synthesis of the included studies. Once the studies had been retrieved from the electronic database search, a thorough evaluation against our predefined inclusion and exclusion criteria was performed to confirm each study's adequacy for inclusion in our review and their relevance. Selection, comparability, and reporting outcome measures were evaluated according to the Newcastle–Ottawa Scale (NOS) [5]. No restriction about the minimum number of studies or level of consistency required for synthesis was applied. For each included manuscript, available information regarding the study design, population, condition (the description of laryngeal features), time from diagnosis to intervention, intervention (method of reduction), outcome and follow-up controls was extracted and stored in an Excel file (Microsoft Corporation, Redmond, WA, USA). Any disagreements were resolved by a discussion among the research team. Appropriate tables were created to summarize the results.

2.5. *Quantitative Analysis*

A meta-analysis approach was applied to compare the results of different arytenoid reduction approaches and the effects of TT on outcomes. Pooled weighted mean differences (WMDs) were estimated using a random-effects model.

A random-effects model was fitted to the data to consider both within- and between-study variability. The amount of heterogeneity, represented by tau^2, was estimated using the restricted maximum-likelihood estimator. The Q-test for heterogeneity and the I^2 statistic were also calculated to assess the presence and magnitude of heterogeneity among the studies. If any amount of heterogeneity was detected ($tau^2 > 0$), a prediction interval for the true outcomes was provided. The Meta-Analysis Online Software 2024 (available at https://metaanalysisonline.com/) was used to perform the quantitative analysis.

3. Results

3.1. *Retrieved Studies and Quality Assessment*

A total of 61 papers was found through title and abstract screening: 20 studies were already retrieved [8,11–28] from the previously published systematic review, while 41 records resulted from the updated literature search of English-language studies through PubMed, Cochrane and Scopus databases (after duplicates were removed). After full-text screening, 48 articles were excluded because they did not match the inclusion criteria. Thirteen studies [11,12,14–17,20,22,24–28] were considered eligible for entering our systematic review. Figure 1 summarizes the study selection process.

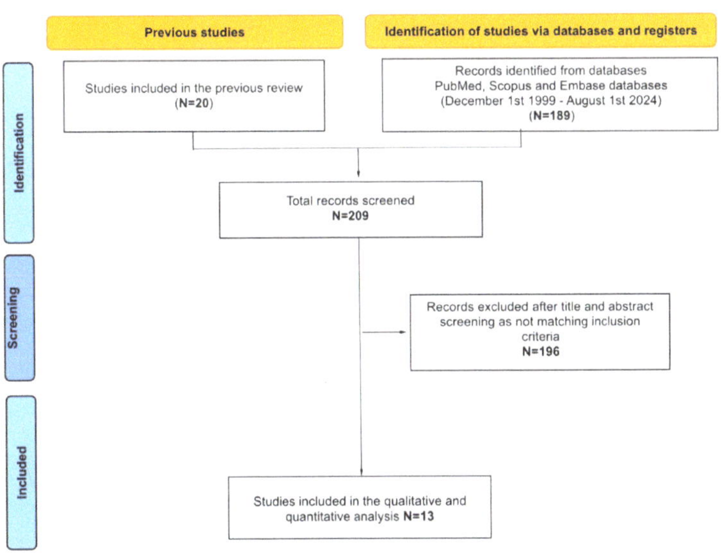

Figure 1. PRISMA diagram from identification to inclusion.

All included studies had adequate relevance to the subject of this review. One investigation was prospective [28] and twelve were retrospective [11,12,14–17,20,22,24–26,28].

According to the NOS, 69.2% of the selected studies scored 5/8 [14–16,20,22–24,27,28], while 31.8% of them scored 4/8 [11,12,17,26].

3.2. Main Features of Included Studies

A total of 361 patients were enrolled; the mean age was 46.95 years, and 53.7% of them were male, as depicted in Table 1.

The most frequent etiology of AS/AD was iatrogenic trauma due to intubation (ranging between 61.76% [20] and 100% [18,22,24,25,28] of the cases), while the second reported cause was laryngeal external blunt trauma (from 15.9% [14] to 28% [28]). A few cases of spontaneous AS/AD were reported [15,16]. Sometimes, AS/AD causes were idiopathic or not recorded [12,14,20]. AS/AD's most commonly reported symptom was dysphonia [11,12,14,16,17,20,22,24–27], followed by dysphagia [14,17,24], and dyspepsia [12,26].

In 50.1% of cases, arytenoids were found to be dislocated on the left side and in 31.6% on the right side. Bilateral arytenoid dislocation (AD) was disclosed in 2.2% of cases. The side of dislocation was unspecified in 16.1% of cases [16,27]. Various classification systems have been reported to categorize the direction of dislocation, including (i) the anterior–posterior classification [11,12,26,27]; (ii) a combined anterior–posterior/medial–lateral classification [16,17,25], which also considers subtypes based on the position of the arytenoid tip [16]; (iii) the anterior–posterior-complex classification [14]; and (iv) the cranio-caudal/medial–lateral classification [15]. Instead, the specific direction of dislocation was not defined by three groups [20,22,24,28].

Fibroscopy was used in 12 out of 13 studies to objectively assess AD/AS. In order to confirm the diagnosis, a computerized tomography scan was performed in 11 out of 13 studies, using high-resolution images and/or 3D reconstructions [11,12,14,15,17,18,20,22,25–28]. Sometimes, laryngeal electromyography (LEMG) was also used [14–16,25,27].

3.3. Treatment and Outcomes

Spontaneous recovery was found in nine AD/AS patients [12,14,15,20,22,24,27]; for all other cases, CR was a first-choice treatment. Rubin [14], Lou [22], Zheng [26], and Cao [20] reported having had to repeat the procedure more than once in refracted patients. In a small percentage of cases (33 out of 361, 9.15%), other surgical treatments (i.e., injection laryngoplasty, botulinum injection, and thyroplasty) were performed alongside CR in order to treat refractory cases, as depicted in Table 1 [14,15,20,27]. TT ranged from 1 to 6223 days, with a mean of 80.9 days (SD 122.9). After treatment, fibroscopy was performed to investigate vocal fold mobility, while voice quality was analyzed through the Voice Handicap Index (VHI), GRBAS scale, and acoustic voice analysis in the majority of studies [11,12,15,20,25–28]. Otherwise, direct questions to patients and/or subjective voice quality questionnaires were administered [11,12]. As depicted in Table 1, voice outcomes were as follows: 68.1% normal, 18.4% improved, 2.7% slightly improved, and 10.8% unchanged. Based on these categories, data were divided into two groups: successful treatment (comprising both normal and improved outcomes) and unsuccessful treatment (including slightly improved and unchanged outcomes). A meta-analysis was then conducted on these dichotomized data, with the findings detailed in the following section.

Table 1. Characteristics and main findings of included studies.

Reference	No. Cases (Sex)	Mean Age in Years ± SD (Range)	Type of AS/AD (No. Cases)	Etiology (No. Cases)	Instrumental Tests	Type of Treatment (No. Cases)	Mean TT in Days ± SD (Range)	Outcome (No. Cases)
Rubin 2005 [14]	63 (24 M, 39 F)	42.5 (18.6)	AD-L (35), AD-R (25) AD-B (3) ant (17) post (32) complex (5) ant -post (3) NR (6)	Intubation (49) External blunt trauma (10) Anesthesia (1) Whiplash (1) Idiopathic (1) NR (1)	Fibro CT LEMG Subjective and objective evaluation of voice quality	SR (2), CR (35), CR + injection laryngoplasty (21), CR + Thyroplasty I (2), Voice therapy (3)	Successful 680.4 ± 1196.3 Unsuccessful 1959.3 ± 2954	N (10) I (31) SI (9) U (5) Lost F-U (6)
Hiramatsu 2010 [15]	12 (8M, 4F)	65 (39–88)	AD-L (8), AD-R (4) Medio-caudal (6) medio-cranial (5) Latero-cranial (1)	Intubation (8) Idiopathic (4)	CT LEMG MPT AVA	SR (2) CR (3) Thyroplasty I (3) Untreated (4)	5.5 ± 6.6	I (3) U (3) Lost F-U (4)
Leelamanit 2012 [16]	29 (8M, 21F)	42.48 (12–77)	AD ant-med (28) AD post-lat (1) Subtypes I (18); II (6); III (4)	Intubation (26) Spontaneous (3)	Fibro LEMG Voice quality of life Patients' global voice quality	CR (29)	5.45 ± 8.26	N (21) I (5) U (3)
Lee 2013 [17]	11 (7M, 4F)	55	AD-L (8) AD-R (3) ant-med (10) post-lat (1)	Intubation (9) External blunt trauma (2)	Fibro CT Subjective and objective evaluation of voice quality	CR (11)	49.8 ± 41.48	N (6) I (5)
Lee 2014 [27]	22 (10M,12F)	36.6	AD ant (16) AD post (6)	Intubation (16) External laryngeal trauma (6)	Fibro CT LEMG AVA VHI	CR (16), SR (1), CR + injection laryngoplasty (4), CR + botulinum (1)	21 (7–6223)	N (18) U (3)
Teng 2014 [11]	12 (8M, 4F)	35 (22–53)	AD-L (5) AD-R (6) AD-B (1) Ant (11) L-ant R-post (1)	Mechanical pressing (3) Traffic accident (6) Punch (2) Stick fighting (1)	Fibro CT VHI MTP	CR (12)	Successful 43.4 ± 34.1 Unsuccessful 157.7 ± 76.1	N (5) I (4) U (3)
Lee 2015 [28]	13 (6M, 7F)	54.1 ± 15.9	AD-L (8) AD-R (5)	Intubation	Fibro CT Subjective and objective evaluation of voice quality	CR (13)	22.2 ± 28.8	N (13)

Table 1. *Cont.*

Reference	No. Cases (Sex)	Mean Age in Years ± SD (Range)	Type of AS/AD (No. Cases)	Etiology (No. Cases)	Instrumental Tests	Type of Treatment (No. Cases)	Mean TT in Days ± SD (Range)	Outcome (No. Cases)
Lou 2016 [12]	35 (21M, 14F)	51.7	AD-L (19) AD-R (16) ant (32) post (3)	Tracheal intubation for surgery (30) Ventilation (3) Gastric tube (2)	Fibro CT VHI MPT	SR (1) CR (34)	17.4 ± 11.7	N (34)
Cao 2016 [20]	34 (24M, 10F)	46.96 ± 18.85	AD-L (20) AD-R (12) AD-B (2)	Intubation (21) Blunt trauma (11) LMA insertion (2)	Fibro CT LEMG GRBAS VHI AVA	SR (1) CR (31) CR + injection laryngoplasty (2)	Successful 18.5 ± 9.5 Unsuccessful 41.9 ± 29.3	N (26) SI (7)
Lou 2017 [22]	28 (18M, 10F)	55 ± 12 (22–76)	AD-L (16) AD-R (12)	Intubation	Fibro CT VHI MPT	SR (1) CR (27)	NR	N (27)
Hung 2018 [24]	14 (6M, 8F)	36.9	AD-L (13) AD-R (1)	Intubation	Fibro	SR (1) CR (13)	Successful 6.2 ± 4.3 Unsuccessful 19 ± 24.1	N (11) U (2)
Wu 2019 [25]	57 (38M, 19F)	47.09 ± 17.82 (15–83)	AD-L (36) AD-R (19) AD-B (2) ant-med (53) post-lat (4)	Intubation (42) Blunt trauma (15)	Fibro CT LEMG VHI GRBAS	CR (57)	NR	N (24) I (15) U (18)
Zheng 2019 [26]	31 (16M, 15F)	50.97 (22–76)	AD-L (18) AD-R (13) ant (22) post (9)	Intubation (31)	Fibro CT VHI GRBAS AVA	CR (31)	20.2 ± 4.19	N (31)

Abbreviations: AD: arytenoid dislocation, AS: arytenoid subluxation; B: bilateral; AVA: acoustic voice analysis; B: bilateral, CR: close reduction, CT: computed tomography, Fibro: fibroscopy, F-U: follow-up, GRBAS: grave, roughness, breathiness, asthenia, strain, HNR: harmonics-to-noise ratio, I: improved, L: left side, MPT: maximum phonation time, N: normal/fully recovered, NOS: Newcastle–Ottawa Scale, NR: not reported, R: right side, SI: slightly improved, SR: spontaneous recovery, SRed: spontaneous reduction, U: unchanged, VF: vocal fold, VHI: voice handicap index.

3.4. Quantitative Analysis

The proportion analysis conducted on general anesthesia (GA) groups [14–17,24,27,28] included a total of seven studies (k = 7), as shown in Figure 2.

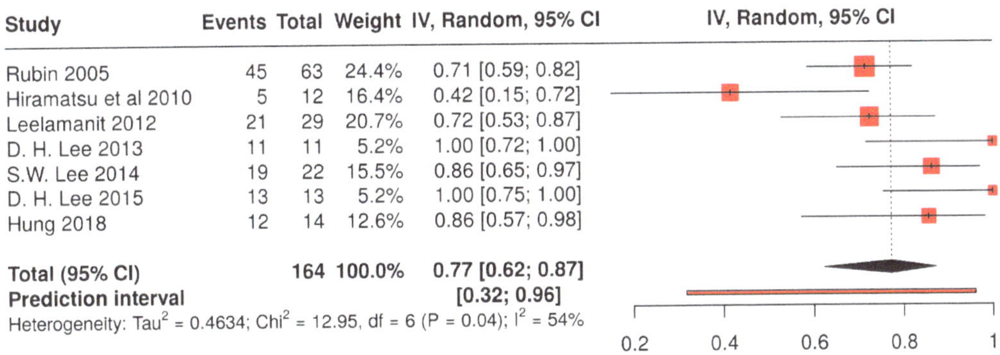

Figure 2. Forest plot showing pooled outcomes of closed reduction under general anesthesia [14–17,24,27,28].

The pooled analysis using a random-effects model resulted in an overall effect size of 0.77 (95% CI: 0.62, 0.87; $p < 0.05$). The second proportion analysis (Figure 3) with six studies on local anesthesia (LA) groups [11,12,20,22,25,26] showed an overall effect estimate of 0.89 (95% CI: 0.70, 0.97; $p < 0.05$).

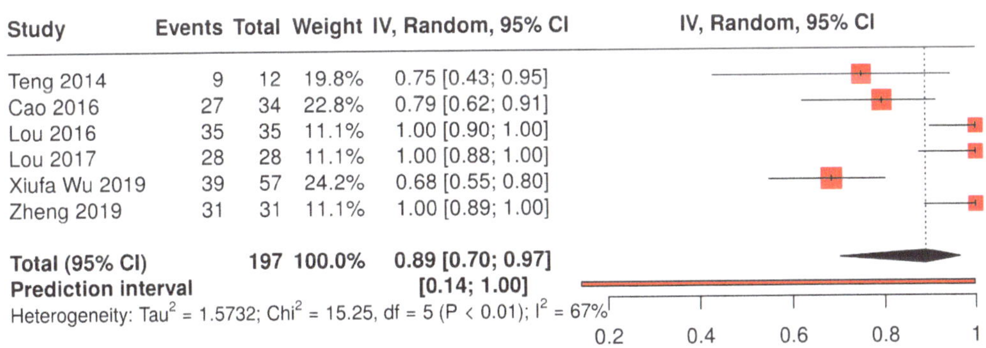

Figure 3. Forest plot showing pooled outcomes of closed reduction under local anesthesia [11,12,20,22,25,26].

In both proportion analyses, a moderate level of heterogeneity was observed among the included studies (54% and 67%, respectively). The Tau^2 values of 1.5732 (GA) and 0.4634 (LA) further suggest some variability in effect sizes. The prediction interval, ranging from 0.14 to 1.00 (GA) and from 0.32 to 0.96 (LA), indicates that while the intervention generally appears beneficial, the effect size could vary across different contexts and potentially include no effect. A total of four studies [11,14,20,24] were included in the TT analysis (Figure 4).

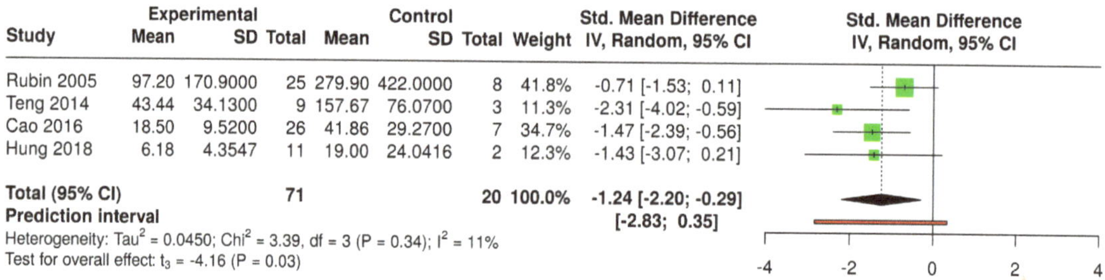

Figure 4. Forest plot showing pooled outcomes of effects of TT on the efficacy of closed reduction [11,14,20,24].

The pooled standardized mean difference using a random-effects model was −1.24 (95% CI: −2.20, −0.29), indicating a statistically significant overall effect favouring the experimental group ($p = 0.03$), meaning that a reduced TT positively affected the treatment outcome. Among the individual studies, two showed significant results: Teng 2014 (−2.31, 95% CI: −4.02, −0.59) and Cao 2016 (−1.47, 95% CI: −2.39, −0.56) [11,16]. In contrast, the studies by Rubin 2005 and Hung 2018 did not reach statistical significance, as their confidence intervals were zero [14,24]. Heterogeneity across studies was low, with an I2 value of 11% and a non-significant χ^2 test for heterogeneity ($p = 0.34$), suggesting that the observed variation in effect sizes was largely due to random errors rather than true differences between studies. The prediction interval, ranging from −2.83 to 0.35, indicates that although the intervention generally favours the experimental group, future studies might observe variability, potentially including null or slightly positive effects.

4. Discussion

AS and AD are often underestimated or misdiagnosed conditions which result in the reduced mobility of the vocal fold and incomplete glottic closure [8]. In this updated systematic review and meta-analysis, 13 studies were included. They focused on the diagnosis, treatment, and TT of AS/AD. Nonetheless, the absence of randomized controlled trials (RCTs) limited this investigation. Moreover, a low quality of available evidence of the selected papers was found: no studies scored more than five out of eight for the NOS score.

Revealing a mean patient age of 46.95 years and a predominance of males (53.7%), the demographic data aligned with the knowledge that AS/AD can affect adults across a wide age range, even though pediatric cases have been reported [29]. The prevalence of iatrogenic trauma, specifically due to intubation, as the most common etiology of AS/AD (ranging from 61.76% to 100% of cases) underscores the clinical challenge of managing airways, especially in critical care or surgical settings. External laryngeal blunt trauma, the second cause, pointed to the vulnerability of the laryngeal apparatus due to physical injury and may partially justify the slightly higher prevalence in males [29]. The presence of spontaneous cases, although few, along with idiopathic causes, highlights the complexity of AS/AD's etiology and the need for thorough diagnostic processes. A notable finding was the higher prevalence of left-sided dislocation (50.1%) over right-sided dislocation (31.6%), with bilateral dislocations being uncommon (2.2%). This asymmetry could suggest an anatomical or biomechanical predisposition for left-sided injuries, possibly related to the direction of endotracheal tube insertion [30]. However, the absence of a standardized classification system complicated the interpretation and comparison of findings across studies, thus limiting our understanding of the condition's nuances and best treatment approaches. The overlapping symptomatology and endoscopic findings between AS/AD and Recurrent Laryngeal Nerve neuropathies can make differential diagnosis a challenge in the absence of adequate professional expertise and complete diagnostic workouts. The use of fibroscopy and computerized tomography scans for AS/AD identification in the included studies, as well as LEMG in some cases, illustrated the multi-modal approach required, in line with existing diagnostic algorithms [5]. Moreover, the assessment of voice quality through the VHI, GRBAS scale, and acoustic voice analysis provided a comprehensive evaluation framework that underscored the need for specialized care and resources to treat AS/AD patients. Given that ultrasound has recently proven to be a valuable non-invasive imaging technique for detecting the abnormal positioning of the cricoarytenoid joint, there is growing interest in future research on its role in AS/AD, which, to date, has been explored in only a single case report [31].

Concerning treatment, all clinical research groups reported CR as a first-choice treatment, performed with different anesthesiological and surgical techniques. In CR under general anesthesia, according to Rubin et al. (2005), anterior dislocations are reduced using a Hollinger laryngoscope, which facilitates direct visualization and access to anterior laryngeal structures, while posterior dislocations are managed with a Miller-3 laryngoscope positioned in the ipsilateral pyriform sinus, providing appropriate leverage and access for a reduction in posteriorly displaced structures [14]. Subsequently, Leelamanit et al. (2012) introduced a reduction technique using two custom-made stainless-steel rods approximately 30 cm long with a 0.3 cm shaft diameter, tapering to a blunt, hooked tip [16]. According to the authors, this method allows for precise manipulation—with one rod stabilizing the vocal process and the other providing rotational force—which is repeatable and tailored to the dislocation's subtype that may be preferable to traditional methods, particularly in resistant cases [16]. According to Cao et al. (2016), CR under local anesthesia begins with the application of a 1% tetracaine spray to the oropharyngeal region, followed by further anesthesia directly to the laryngeal surface via an indirect laryngoscope. With the patient phonating the vowel sound "[i:]", the surgeon uses laryngeal forceps to grasp the posterior–lateral surface of the dislocated arytenoid cartilage and applies gentle rotational force in an antero-upward direction to guide the arytenoid back into position [20]. It was also observed that CR under local anesthesia usually had to be repeated to achieve reduction [20,22,26]. However, there is still controversy regarding the optimal timing for performing closed reduction in order to obtain the best treatment outcome. Previously, relatively stable treatment outcomes and short recovery duration were shown in patients treated between the 13th and 26th day after AD occurrence, with a TT of less than 21 days that seemed to be predictive of the final outcome. According to Lou et al. (2017) [22], after this time, patients may be refractory, and even if a second treatment could be proposed, recovery may only be partial, probably due to the fibrosis caused by mechanical injury that increases the joint's stiffness, affecting the therapeutic effects of the CR [12]. Sataloff et al. [32] found stable and good treatment outcomes performing CR within 10 weeks after AS or AD, although, in some cases, treatments performed years after the dislocation were also effective [14]. Our investigation revealed that the time from diagnosis to treatment ranged between 1 and 6223 days, with a mean of 80.9 days (SD 122.9). It emerged that a relevant percentage of patients (68.1%) gained full recovery, with their voices returning to their pre-injury quality with affected vocal folds moving normally. Patients who were refractory or felt embarrassed by their voices underwent secondary surgery [14,15,20,27]. In these cases, vocal fold injection was preferred to thyroplasty and voice rehabilitation therapy, as shown in Table 1. Consequently, an early, closed-reduction treatment might improve the success rate and avoid secondary interventions.

The quantitative analysis of the reports supported the qualitative evidence mentioned above. In particular, these findings indicated a high success rate with CR under both general (success rate 77%, CI from 62% to 87%) and local anesthesia (success rate 89%, CI from 70%

to 97%). The TT analysis revealed a significant association between reduced time intervals and improved outcomes in AD/AS management. With the majority of standardized mean differences being negative across the four included studies, the estimated average standardized mean difference of −1.24 underscores the clinical significance of timely intervention. These findings emphasize the importance of prioritizing early treatment initiation to optimize patient outcomes and minimize the potential complications associated with delayed intervention. However, further research is warranted to elucidate the optimal timing for treatment initiation and to better understand the underlying mechanisms driving this observed association. None of the analyses showed significant asymmetry in the funnel plot, and the studies included seemed to be reliable as there were no outliers or influential studies.

This systematic review and meta-analysis, while providing valuable insights into the treatment of AS and AD, were characterized by some limitations. The exclusion of non-English language studies may have introduced selection bias, potentially omitting relevant findings published in other languages, while a recent meta-epidemiological study pointed out that the omission of non-English research in the language literature did not significantly change the size or direction of effect estimates or statistical significance in systematic reviews and meta-analysis [33]. Furthermore, the choice of focused search terms, specifically "arytenoid dislocation" and "arytenoid subluxation", was intended to ensure the relevance and specificity of the included studies. However, this conservative strategy might have excluded studies addressing related conditions (e.g., vocal fold immobility) that could provide indirect insights into AS/AD management. Moreover, the absence of RCTs and the overall moderate-to-low quality of the studies (NOS 5/8) highlighted the importance of the findings' careful interpretation. Finally, the variability among the studies underscores the crucial need for high-quality, prospective research on this topic. This heterogeneity, while reflecting real-world clinical practice, complicates the process of drawing firm conclusions about the optimal timing and approach for treating AS/AD. Although our analysis supported the hypothesis that a reduced TT interval may be beneficial, the variability in outcomes across the studies suggested that individual patient factors and specific treatment contexts could play crucial roles in determining success. Despite these limitations, this review has several strengths that contribute to its value in the field. It represents one of the most comprehensive efforts to synthesize the available evidence about AS/AD treatment, incorporating a wide range of studies and treatment outcomes. The methodological rigour of our systematic review protocol, adherence to PRISMA guidelines, and the use of the NOS for quality assessment ensure that our analysis is systematic and reproducible. This systematic review and meta-analysis improve our understanding of the optimal timing and treatment modalities for AD/AS. It offers a foundation for future research and clinical practice, emphasizing the importance of early and tailored interventions.

5. Conclusions

According to the available evidence, CR appeared to be the preferred treatment for AS/AD, with a high success rate under both general and local anesthesia. A reduced TT seemed to significantly impact recovery from the disease and could be considered a prognostic factor for treatment success. However, given the intrinsic limitations of the available studies on AS/AD, as discussed above, the results of this meta-analysis should not be considered conclusive. Specifically, further data from prospective clinical trials, possibly in a multi-centric setting, are advocated to obtain stronger evidence on the treatment outcomes of AS/AD.

Author Contributions: Conceptualization, A.L.; methodology, A.F.; formal analysis, A.F. and L.F.; investigation, V.C. and G.B.; resources V.C. and G.B.; data curation V.C. and G.B.; statistical analysis, A.F., P.B. and L.V.; writing—original draft preparation, A.F., V.C. and G.B.; writing—review and editing, V.C., G.M., G.B., A.F., L.F., E.G., C.d.F. and A.L.; visualization, all authors; supervision, G.M., C.d.F., L.V., E.G. and A.L.; funding acquisition, not applicable. All authors have read and agreed to the published version of the manuscript.

Funding: Università degli Studi di Padova, Grant/Award Number: DOR2399707/23 (G. Marioni).

Institutional Review Board Statement: Not applicable.

Informed Consent Statement: Not applicable.

Data Availability Statement: Data will be made available on request by the corresponding author.

Acknowledgments: The authors thank Alison Garside for correcting the English version of this paper.

Conflicts of Interest: The authors declare no conflicts of interest.

References

1. Storck, C.; Juergens, P.; Fischer, C.; Wolfensberger, M.; Honegger, F.; Sorantin, E.; Friedrich, G.; Gugatschka, M. Biomechanics of the cricoarytenoid joint: Three-dimensional imaging and vector analysis. *J. Voice* **2010**, *25*, 406–410. [CrossRef] [PubMed]
2. Wang, R.C. Three-dimensional analysis of cricoarytenoid joint motion. *Laryngoscope* **1998**, *108* (Suppl. S86), 1–17. [CrossRef] [PubMed]
3. Paulsen, F.; Jungmann, K.; Thale, A.; Tillmann, B. The joint capsule of the cricoarytenoid joint: Biomechanical and clinical aspects. *Laryngorhinootologie* **2000**, *79*, 412–415. [CrossRef] [PubMed]
4. Kasperbauer, J.L. A biomechanical study of the human cricoarytenoid joint. *Laryngoscope* **1998**, *108*, 1704–1711. [CrossRef] [PubMed]
5. Frosolini, A.; Marioni, G.; Maiolino, L.; de Filippis, C.; Lovato, A. Current management of arytenoid subluxation and dislocation. *Eur. Arch. Otorhinolaryngol.* **2020**, *277*, 2977–2986. [CrossRef] [PubMed]
6. Alalyani, N.S.; Alhedaithy, A.A.; Alshammari, H.K.; AlHajress, R.I.; Alelyani, R.H.; Alshammari, M.F.; Alhalafi, A.H.; Alharbi, A.; Aldabal, N. Incidence and Risk Factors of Arytenoid Dislocation Following Endotracheal Intubation: A Systematic Review and Meta-Analysis. *Cureus* **2024**, *16*, e67917. [CrossRef]
7. Yan, W.Q.; Li, C.; Chen, Z. Delayed diagnosis of arytenoid cartilage dislocation after tracheal intubation in the intensive care unit: A case report. *World J. Clin. Cases* **2022**, *10*, 5119–5123. [CrossRef] [PubMed]
8. Mallon, A.S.; Portnoy, J.E.; Landrum, T.; Sataloff, R.T. Pediatric arytenoid dislocation: Diagnosis and treatment. *J. Voice* **2014**, *28*, 115–122. [CrossRef] [PubMed]
9. Paulsen, F.P.; Jungmann, K.; Tillmann, B.N. The cricoarytenoid joint capsule and its relevance to endotracheal intubation. *Anesth. Analg.* **2000**, *90*, 180–185. [CrossRef] [PubMed]
10. Liu, K.; Hu, H.; Lu, Y.; Yu, Z. A novel five-step reduction technique of arytenoid dislocation. *Laryngoscope* **2024**, *134*, 1744–1748. [CrossRef]
11. Teng, Y.; Wang, H.E.; Lin, Z. Arytenoid cartilage dislocation from external blunt laryngeal trauma: Evaluation and therapy without laryngeal electromyography. *Med. Sci. Monit.* **2014**, *20*, 1496–1502. [CrossRef] [PubMed]
12. Lou, Z.; Lin, Z. The appropriate time for closed reduction using local anesthesia in arytenoid dislocation caused by intubation: A clinical research. *Acta Otolaryngol.* **2017**, *137*, 331–336. [CrossRef] [PubMed]
13. Wang, Z.; Liu, Q. A comparative study on the close reduction of arytenoid dislocation under indirect and direct laryngoscope. *J. Huazhong Univ. Sci. Technolog. Med. Sci.* **2002**, *22*, 375–377. [CrossRef] [PubMed]
14. Rubin, A.D.; Hawkshaw, M.J.; Moyer, C.A.; Dean, C.M.; Sataloff, R.T. Arytenoid cartilage dislocation: A 20-year experience. *J. Voice* **2005**, *19*, 687–701. [CrossRef] [PubMed]
15. Hiramatsu, H.; Tokashiki, R.; Kitamura, M.; Motohashi, R.; Tsukahara, K.; Suzuki, M. New approach to diagnose arytenoid dislocation and subluxation using three-dimensional computed tomography. *Eur. Arch. Otorhinolaryngol.* **2010**, *267*, 1893–1903. [CrossRef] [PubMed]
16. Leelamanit, V.; Sinkijcharoenchai, W. A promising new technique for closed reduction of arytenoid dislocation. *J. Laryngol. Otol.* **2012**, *126*, 168–174. [CrossRef] [PubMed]
17. Lee, D.H.; Yoon, T.M.; Lee, J.K.; Lim, S.C. Treatment outcomes of closed reduction of arytenoid dislocation. *Acta Otolaryngol.* **2013**, *133*, 518–522. [CrossRef] [PubMed]

18. Shen, L.; Wang, W.T.; Yu, X.R.; Zhang, X.H.; Huang, Y.G. Evaluation of risk factors for arytenoid dislocation after endotracheal intubation: A retrospective case-control study. *Chin. Med. Sci. J.* **2014**, *29*, 221–224. [CrossRef]
19. Tan, P.H.; Hung, K.C.; Hsieh, S.W.; Chen, T.B.; Liu, P.H.; Chen, W.H. Large-bore calibrating orogastric tube and arytenoid dislocation: A retrospective study. *Br. J. Anaesth.* **2016**, *116*, 296–298. [CrossRef] [PubMed]
20. Cao, L.; Wu, X.; Mao, W.; Hayes, C.; Wei, C. Closed reduction for arytenoid dislocation under local anesthesia. *Acta Otolaryngol.* **2016**, *136*, 812–818. [CrossRef] [PubMed]
21. Tsuru, S.; Wakimoto, M.; Iritakenishi, T.; Ogawa, M.; Hayashi, Y. Cardiovascular operation: A significant risk factor of arytenoid cartilage dislocation/subluxation after anesthesia. *Ann. Card. Anaesth.* **2017**, *20*, 309–312. [CrossRef]
22. Lou, Z.; Yu, X.; Li, Y.; Duan, H.; Zhang, P.; Lin, Z. BMI may be the risk factor for arytenoid dislocation caused by endotracheal intubation: A retrospective case-control study. *J. Voice* **2018**, *32*, 221–225. [CrossRef] [PubMed]
23. Wu, L.; Shen, L.; Zhang, Y.; Zhang, X.; Huang, Y. Association between the use of a stylet in endotracheal intubation and postoperative arytenoid dislocation: A case-control study. *BMC Anesthesiol.* **2018**, *18*, 59. [CrossRef]
24. Hung, K.C.; Chen, Y.T.; Chen, J.Y.; Kuo, C.Y.; Wu, S.C.; Chiang, M.H.; Lan, K.M.; Wang, L.K.; Sun, C.K. Clinical characteristics of arytenoid dislocation in patients undergoing bariatric/metabolic surgery: A STROBE-compliant retrospective study. *Medicine* **2019**, *98*, e15318. [CrossRef] [PubMed]
25. Wu, X.; Mao, W.; Zhang, J.; Wei, C. Treatment outcomes of arytenoid dislocation by closed reduction: A multidimensional evaluation. *J. Voice* **2021**, *35*, 463–467. [CrossRef]
26. Zheng, T.; Lou, Z.; Li, X.; Teng, Y.; Li, Y.; Lin, X.; Lin, Z. Regularity of voice recovery and arytenoid motion after closed reduction in patients with arytenoid dislocation: A self-controlled clinical study. *Acta Otolaryngol.* **2020**, *140*, 72–78. [CrossRef]
27. Lee, S.W.; Park, K.N.; Welham, N.V. Clinical features and surgical outcomes following closed reduction of arytenoid dislocation. *JAMA Otolaryngol. Head Neck Surg.* **2014**, *140*, 1045–1050. [CrossRef]
28. Lee, D.H.; Yoon, T.M.; Lee, J.K.; Lim, S.C. Clinical characteristics of arytenoid dislocation after endotracheal intubation. *J. Craniofac. Surg.* **2015**, *26*, 1358–1360. [CrossRef] [PubMed]
29. Gabriele, G.; Nigri, A.; Pini, N.; Carangelo, B.R.; Cascino, F.; Fantozzi, V.; Funaioli, F.; Luglietto, D.; Gennaro, P. COVID-19 pandemic: The impact of Italian lockdown on maxillofacial trauma incidence in southern Tuscany. *Ann. Ital. Chir.* **2022**, *92*, 135–139. [PubMed]
30. Xu, X.; Wang, Y.; Wang, J.; Reiss, J.F.; Zhou, L.; Jiang, J.J.; Zhuang, P. Quantitative measurement of the three-dimensional structure of the vocal folds and its application in identifying the type of cricoarytenoid joint dislocation. *J. Voice* **2019**, *33*, 611–619. [CrossRef] [PubMed]
31. Yang, N.; Hua, Z.; Gong, X.; Ma, H. Bedside ultrasound imaging and management of arytenoid cartilage dislocation after tracheal intubation: A case report. *Asian J. Surg.* **2024**, *47*, 4452–4453. [CrossRef]
32. Sataloff, R.T. Arytenoid dislocation: Techniques of surgical reduction. *Oper. Tech. Otolaryngol. Head Neck Surg.* **1998**, *9*, 196–202. [CrossRef]
33. Nussbaumer-Streit, B.; Klerings, I.; Dobrescu, A.I.; Persad, E.; Stevens, A.; Garritty, C.; Kamel, C.; Affengruber, L.; King, V.J.; Gartlehner, G. Excluding non-English publications from evidence-syntheses did not change conclusions: A meta-epidemiological study. *J. Clin. Epidemiol.* **2020**, *118*, 42–54. [CrossRef] [PubMed]

medicina

MDPI

Systematic Review

Effect of the BiZact™ Low-Temperature Dissecting Device on Intra- and Postoperative Morbidities Related to Tonsillectomy—A Systematic Review and Meta-Analysis

Yun Jin Kang [1], Gulnaz Stybayeva [2] and Se Hwan Hwang [3,*]

1 Department of Otorhinolaryngology-Head and Neck Surgery, Soonchunhyang University College of Medicine, Cheonan 14584, Republic of Korea; savie87@gmail.com
2 Department of Physiology and Biomedical Engineering, Mayo Clinic, Rochester, MN 55905, USA; stybayeva.gulnaz@mayo.edu
3 Department of Otolaryngology-Head and Neck Surgery, Bucheon St. Mary's Hospital, College of Medicine, The Catholic University of Korea, Seoul 06591, Republic of Korea
* Correspondence: yellobird@catholic.ac.kr; Tel.: +82-32-340-7044

Abstract: *Background and Objectives*: We investigated the effects of using a BiZact™ device for tonsillectomy on operating time, intraoperative blood loss, postoperative bleeding rate, and pain through a meta-analysis of the relevant literature. *Materials and Methods*: We reviewed studies retrieved from the databases of PubMed, SCOPUS, Google Scholar, Embase, Web of Science, and Cochrane up to March 2024. The results were analyzed following PRISMA guidelines. Six studies that compared the outcomes of patients receiving perioperative BiZact™ tonsillectomy with those in control groups (cold steel dissection or bipolar tonsillectomy) were included for this analysis of the outcomes, which included intraoperative bleeding and time, postoperative pain, and frequency of postoperative bleeding. *Results*: The operative time (SMD −11.5985, 95%CI [−20.3326; −2.8644], I^2 = 99.5%) in the treatment group was significantly reduced compared to the control group. However, BiZact™ showed no significant efficacy in reducing intraoperative bleeding when compared with the control group (SMD −0.0480, 95%CI [−1.8200; 1.7240], I^2 = 98.6%). Postoperative pain on day 1 (SMD −0.0885, 95%CI [−0.4368; 0.2598], I^2 = 98.9%), day 3 (SMD −0.2118, 95%CI [−0.6110; 0.1873], I^2 = 99.5%), and later than day 7 (SMD 0.0924, 95%CI [−0.2491; 0.4338], I^2 = 98.6%) in the treatment group was not significantly reduced relative to the control group. When compared to the control group, BiZact™ did not reduce the incidence of secondary postoperative bleeding control in the operation room (OR 0.5711, 95%CI [0.2476; 1.3173], I^2 = 32.1%), primary bleeding (OR 0.4514, 95%CI [0.0568; 3.5894], I^2 = 0.0%), or all postoperative bleeding events (OR 0.8117, 95%CI [0.5796; 1.1368], I^2 = 26.3%). *Conclusions*: This study demonstrated that using the BiZact™ device for tonsillectomy significantly decreased the operative time but could not effectively reduce intraoperative bleeding or postoperative pain and bleeding.

Keywords: tonsillectomy; pain; adverse effect; meta-analysis

1. Introduction

Tonsillectomy is one of the most common surgeries worldwide [1,2]. Postoperative pain is a major concern following tonsillectomy. Although it has a relatively short operative time, it may involve postoperative bleeding and pain, along with a delayed return to a normal diet [3]. Post-tonsillectomy bleeding and pain remain an important issue [4]. The optimal surgical method and surgical device have yet to be determined and remain an active area of study [5]. Post-tonsillectomy pain intensity is dependent on the type of tonsillectomy, intra- and postoperative medications, and tissue damage from bleeding control [6–8]. Cold steel dissection, a traditional tonsillectomy method, uses instruments to remove the palatine tonsil and ligate the blood vessels with sutures [5,9]. Hot dissection with electro-cauterization, coblation, or a diathermia scissor is also widely used [1]. Tonsillectomy using electro-cauterization has the advantage of achieving reductions in surgical time and intraoperative bleeding, but there is also a risk of post-tonsillectomy pain or bleeding [10]. About 1.3–20% of patients reported post-tonsillectomy bleeding [11].

The BIZact™ (Medtronic, Mansfield, MA, USA) is a new surgical device for vessel sealing that takes continuous measurements of tissue impedance, and which received approval in 2016 [12,13]. BiZact™ consists of a 12 cm shaft and a curved jaw that provides easy access to the tonsillar bed [12]. When the tissue is sufficiently sealed between the jaws, an acoustic signal is generated and the tissue is cut [12]. Tissue damage is minimized by delivering minimal bipolar energy to the remaining tissues around the tonsil [13]. A major feature is the reduction in thermal spread to the surrounding tissues [12]. Tonsillectomy using this device is ultimately a safe surgery with a short surgical time and relatively short learning curve [14].

There have been various studies confirming the effectiveness of BiZact™ on pediatric tonsillectomies [14–17], and its effectiveness has been proven in comparison to LigaSure™ [18]. However, it involves a higher cost than using another bipolar device for tonsillectomy, and there is no statistical certainty that patient morbidity will be reduced [15,16]. There has been no meta-analysis that comprehensively compares and analyzes these pros and cons. To our knowledge, this is the first meta-analysis comparing tonsillectomy using BiZact™ with cold steel dissection or bipolar tonsillectomy in terms of operating time, intraoperative blood loss, and postoperative bleeding rate and pain.

2. Materials and Methods

The Preferred Reporting Items Guidelines for Systematic Review and Meta-Analysis were followed when conducting this systematic review and meta-analysis [19]. This study protocol was prospectively registered in the Open Science Framework as follows: https://osf.io/uxv7p/ (accessed on 1 April 2024).

2.1. Search Strategy and Study Selection

The Population, Intervention, Comparison, Outcomes, and Study (PICOS) details were as follows: (1) Population: patients who underwent tonsillectomy. (2) Intervention: tonsillectomy using the BiZact™ device. (3) Comparison: a bipolar tonsillectomy or cold steel dissection. (4) Outcomes: operative time, intraoperative bleeding, postoperative pain grading, and incidence of postoperative bleeding. (5) Study design: prospective or retrospective study. Clinical studies published prior to March of 2024 were identified from Pubmed, SCOPUS, Google Scholar, Embase, Web of Science, and the Cochrane Register of Controlled Trials. The following key search terms were used: 'bizact', 'tonsillectomy', 'adenotonsillectomy', 'vessel sealing devices', 'pain', 'operative time', and 'bleeding'.

The database search proceeded with the aid of a librarian with more than 10 years of experience, and the authors additionally searched the references listed in the retrieved articles to ensure that there were no missing reports. Two independent reviewers (YJK and SHH) screened all abstracts and titles for the candidate studies and discounted the studies not associated with tonsillectomy using a BiZact™ device. The full texts of potentially relevant studies were used if the decision regarding inclusion could not be made from the abstract alone. In the case of differing opinions, inclusion or exclusion was decided by discussion with a third reviewer (GS). Studies that satisfied the next inclusion criteria were considered to be eligible for review: trials that studied patients undergoing tonsillectomy using the BiZact™ device. We did not include patients who underwent concomitant procedures along with tonsillectomy, such as sleep surgery. Studies were also excluded from the analysis if the outcomes of interest were not clearly provided with quantifiable data, or if it was impossible to evaluate the appropriate data from the published results. Figure 1 summarizes the search strategy used to identify the studies selected for the meta-analysis [1,5,12,20–22].

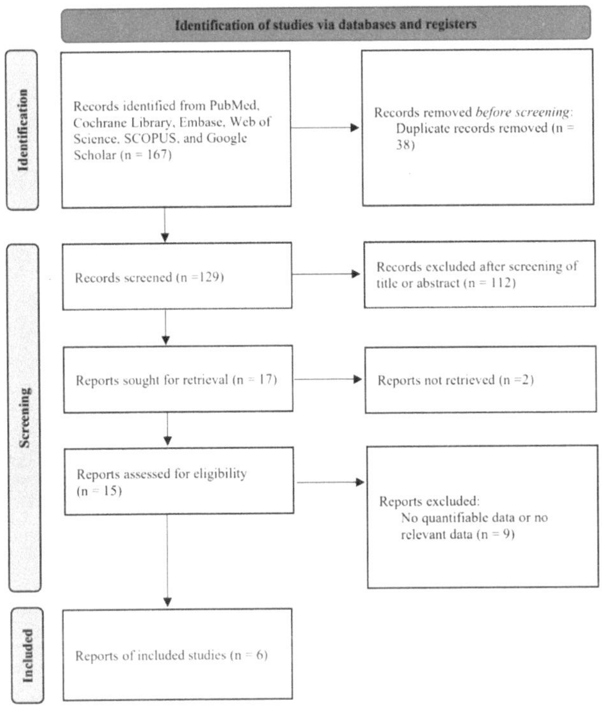

Figure 1. Study selection diagram.

2.2. *Data Extraction and Risk of Bias Assessment*

Data from eligible studies were extracted using standardized forms [23]. The analyzed outcomes were as follows: intraoperative bleeding (grading or amount), operative time, postoperative pain grading reported by patients, and incidence of postoperative bleeding (total bleeding event, primary bleeding (in 24 h after tonsillectomy), bleeding control in operation room). These outcomes were compared between the treatment group and the control group (patients that used no treatment or saline injection) during the perioperative period. From the studies marked for inclusion, we selected data regarding patient number, pain grading scale, operative time, amount of intraoperative bleeding, incidence of postoperative bleeding, and the *p*-value, which was reported in the form of a comparison between the treatment group and the control group. This was conducted to determine the influence of BiZact™ on intra- and postoperative morbidities.

2.3. *Analyses for Statistics*

The statistical analysis of the included studies was conducted using the R-4.3.1 program (R Software Foundation, Vienna, Austria). For quantitative variables, the meta-analysis was conducted using the mean difference (MD) or standardized mean difference (SMD). The SMD was adopted as a summary statistic to standardize the results of the studies to an equal scale when the studies measured the equal outcome but assessed it in various methods. In the incidence of postoperative bleeding, the odds ratio (OR) was calculated. Heterogeneity was calculated using the I^2 test, which describes the rate of variation across studies that can be attributed to heterogeneity rather than probabilistic chance. The measure ranges from 0 (no heterogeneity) to 100 (maximum heterogeneity). All results were reported with 95% confidence intervals (CI), and all *p*-values were two-tailed. When significant heterogeneity among outcomes was found (defined as $I^2 > 50$), the random-effects model was used as described by DerSimonian–Laird. This model assumes that the true treatment effects in individual studies may be different from one another, and that these are normally distributed.

Subgroup analysis was also performed. Those outcomes that did not present a significant level of heterogeneity ($I^2 < 50$) were analyzed with the fixed-effects model. The fixed-effects model uses the inverse variance approach, and it is assumed that all studies come from a common population.

We used a funnel plot and Egger's test concurrently to identify potential publication bias. We also used Duval and Tweedie's trim and fill to compensate for the summed effect size with respect to publication bias. Moreover, to estimate the effect of each individual study in the overall meta-analysis results, sensitivity analyses were conducted. These analyses were performed by repeating the meta-analyses while omitting a different study each time.

3. Results

In total, six studies with 1880 participants were included and reviewed for this meta-analysis. The study characteristics are presented in Table 1 and the results of the bias evaluations are presented in Supplementary Tables S1 and S2.

Table 1. Summary of included studies.

Study	Study Design	Nation	Total Number of Patients (*n*)	Sex (Female/Male)	Age of Patients (Years, Mean ± Standardized Deviation or Range)	Comparison	Outcomes
Besser (2022) [20]	A single-center, randomized, self-controlled trial	Austria	48	11/17	24.3 ± 6.7	BiZact™ tonsillectomy on one tonsil side versus cold steel dissection tonsillectomy on another side	Operative time, intraoperative bleeding, and postoperative bleeding incidence
Falz (2023) [12]	Retrospective case–control study	Germany	183	51/132	28.3 ± 8.9	Patient with BiZact™ versus cold steel dissection tonsillectomy	Operative time, intraoperative bleeding, postoperative pain, and postoperative bleeding incidence
Yildirim (2023) [22]	Prospective case–control study	Turkey	128	61/67	8.2 (5–14)	Patient with BiZact™ versus bipolar tonsillectomy	Operative time, intraoperative bleeding, and postoperative pain
Manhein (2023) [1]	Prospective, randomized, partly double-blinded study	Norway	65	28/37	25 ± 4.9	Patient with BiZact™ versus bipolar tonsillectomy (conventional non-disposable diathermic scissor)	Operative time, intraoperative bleeding, postoperative pain, and postoperative bleeding incidence
Saleem (2022) [21]	A comparative study using non-probability purposive sampling	India	100	46/54	6–21	Patient with BiZact™ versus cold steel dissection tonsillectomy	Operative time, intraoperative bleeding, and postoperative pain
Chuang (2024) [5]	Retrospective single-surgeon cohort study	Austria	1356	668/688	13.3 (2–61)	Patient with BiZact™ versus bipolar tonsillectomy	Postoperative bleeding incidence

3.1. Effect of BiZact™ Tonsillectomy on Intraoperative Time and Bleeding Compared with the Control Group

The BiZact™ device was demonstrated to be effective in reducing intraoperative time when compared with the control group (MD −11.5985 min, 95%CI [−20.3326; −2.8644], I^2 = 99.5%), but it could not reduce intraoperative bleeding (SMD −0.0480, 95%CI [−1.8200; 1.7240], I^2 = 98.6%) (Figure 2).

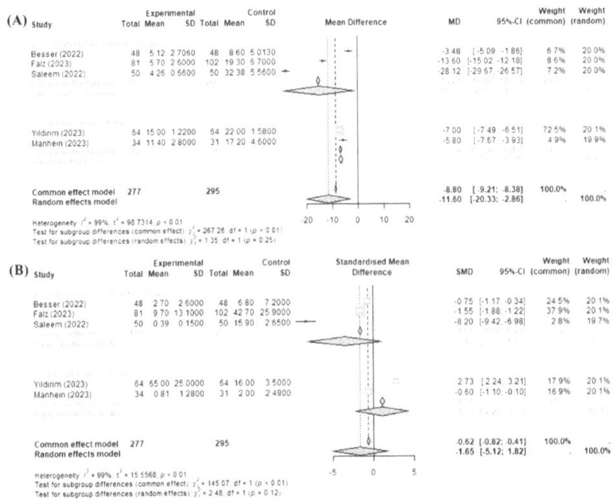

Figure 2. BiZact™ tonsillectomy versus conventional tonsillectomy: (**A**) mean difference in operative time and (**B**) standardized mean difference in intraoperative bleeding. SD: standardized deviation, MD: mean difference, CI: confidence index, SMD: standardized mean difference.

Significant inter-study heterogeneity ($I^2 > 50\%$) was found for the above outcomes. The overall analysis did not consider the particular definition of the control group (bipolar tonsillectomy or cold steel dissection). This omission is reflected in the high heterogeneity (more than 50%) of the results obtained by all studies. In the subgroup analysis of the operative time compared to those of cold steel dissection and bipolar tonsillectomy, operative time was improved with the BiZact™ device (compared to cold steel dissection: MD −15.0662, 95%CI [−29.0798; −1.0526]; compared to bipolar tonsillectomy: MD −6.7545, 95%CI [−7.7033; −5.8058]). By contrast, in the subgroup analysis of operative bleeding compared to those of cold steel dissection and bipolar tonsillectomy, bleeding risk was not improved with the BiZact™ device in any comparison (compared to cold steel dissection: SMD −3.4671, 95%CI [−8.0626; 1.1284]; compared to bipolar tonsillectomy: SMD 1.0637, 95%CI [−2.2006; 4.3281]).

3.2. *Effect of BiZact™ Tonsillectomy on Pain Grading Compared with the Control Group*

Tonsillectomy using BiZact™ did not show a significant effect on postoperative pain on day 1 (SMD −0.0885, 95%CI [−0.4368; 0.2598], $I^2 = 98.9\%$), day 3 (SMD −0.2118, 95%CI [−0.6110; 0.1873], $I^2 = 99.5\%$), and later than day 7 (SMD 0.0924, 95%CI [−0.2491; 0.4338], $I^2 = 98.6\%$) when compared with the control group (Figure 3).

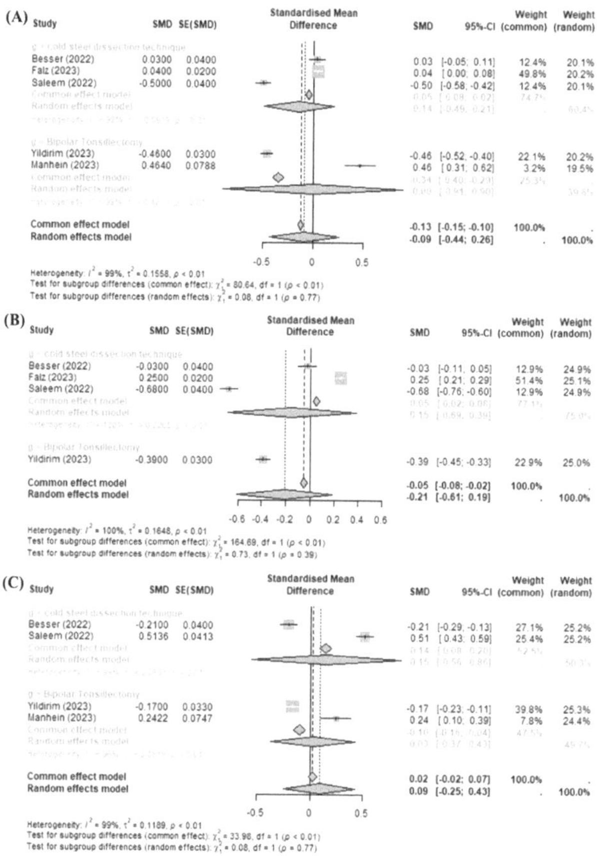

Figure 3. BiZact™ tonsillectomy versus conventional tonsillectomy: standard mean difference in postoperative pain score on (**A**) day 1, (**B**) day 2, and (**C**) later than day 7. SMD: standardized mean difference, SE: standard error, CI: confidence index.

Significant inter-study heterogeneity ($I^2 > 50\%$) was found at the above outcomes. In the subgroup analysis of post-tonsillectomy pain compared to cold steel dissection, the pain score was not improved with the BiZact™ device in any time period of postoperative follow-up (day 1 (SMD −0.1426, 95%CI [−0.4914; 0.2063]), day 3 (SMD −0.1526, 95%CI [−0.6926; 0.3873]), and later than day 7 (SMD 0.1517, 95%CI [−0.5574; 0.8608])). However, compared to bipolar tonsillectomy, the BiZact™ device significantly reduced postoperative pain on day 3 (SMD −0.3900, 95%CI [−0.4488; −0.3312]); there were no significant differences in postoperative pain on day 1 (SMD −0.0009, 95%CI [−0.9064; 0.9046]) or later than day 7 (SMD 0.0307, 95%CI [−0.3732; 0.4345]).

3.3. *Effect of BiZact™ Tonsillectomy on the Incidence of Postoperative Bleeding Compared with the Control Group*

The BiZact™ device did not significantly reduce the incidence of postoperative bleeding control in the operation room (OR 0.5711, 95%CI [0.2476; 1.3173], $I^2 = 32.1\%$), primary bleeding (OR 0.4514, 95%CI [0.0568; 3.5894], $I^2 = 0.0\%$), or all postoperative bleeding events (OR 0.8117, 95%CI [0.5796; 1.1368], $I^2 = 26.3\%$) compared to the control group (Figure 4).

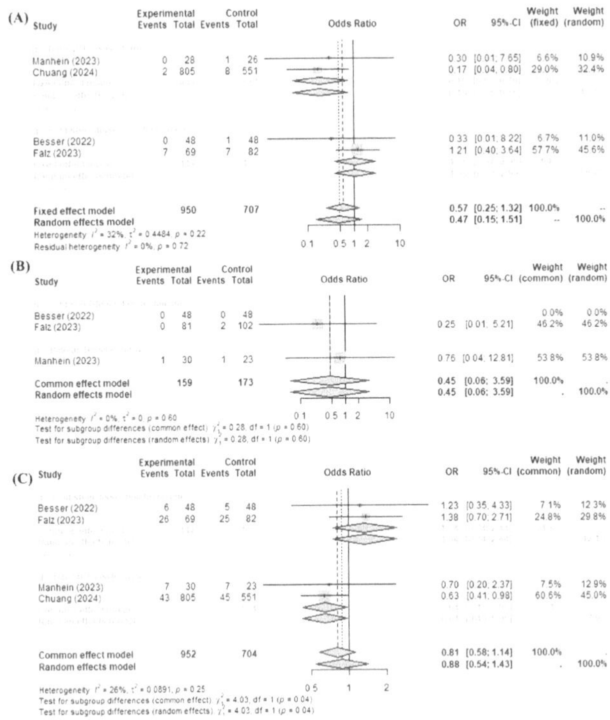

Figure 4. BiZact™ tonsillectomy versus conventional tonsillectomy: odds ratios of (**A**) incidence of postoperative bleeding control in operation room, (**B**) primary bleeding, and (**C**) all postoperative bleeding events. OR: odds ratio, CI: confidence index.

In the subgroup analysis of post-tonsillectomy pain compared to cold steel dissection, the BiZact™ device was not found to significantly reduce the incidence of postoperative bleeding control in the operation room (OR 1.0553, 95%CI [0.3725; 2.9899]), primary bleeding (OR 0.2466, 95%CI [0.0117; 5.2096]), or all postoperative bleeding events (OR 1.3435, 95%CI [0.7400; 2.4391]). Interestingly, the BiZact™ device significantly reduced the incidence of postoperative bleeding control in the operation room (OR 0.1879, 95%CI [0.0463; 0.7629]) and all postoperative bleeding events (OR 0.6410, 95%CI [0.4262; 0.9641]), aside from primary bleeding (OR 0.7586, 95%CI [0.0449; 12.8123]), when compared to bipolar tonsillectomy.

3.4. Sensitivity Analysis

A sensitivity analysis was performed by excluding individual studies from the meta-analysis one by one. No one study was found to significantly impact the overall trend.

4. Discussion

In this study, we compared the effectiveness of the new BiZact™ tonsillectomy device with cold steel dissection or bipolar tonsillectomy for the first time. Tonsillectomy using the BiZact™ device was shown to involve a significantly reduced intraoperative time compared to the control group. However, its effectiveness in reducing intraoperative bleeding compared with the control group was not significant. Post-tonsillectomy pain did not significantly decrease compared to the control group on day 1, day 3, or later than day 7. Lastly, compared to the control group, BiZact™ involved significantly less post-tonsillectomy bleeding.

We confirmed that the intraoperative time for tonsillectomy using BiZact™ was significantly shorter than that for the control group, and previous studies also confirmed that the surgery time was shorter than those of cold steel dissection, bipolar radiofrequency, or other tonsillectomy devices [15,16,24]. Tonsillectomy using bipolar cauterization takes an average of 15 to 20 min, but that using the BiZact™ device is reported to take an average of 4 to 7.5 min [12,14,15,21,24–26].

Our results report that the BiZact™ device did not significantly reduce bleeding risk during or after tonsillectomy. BiZact™ can reduce tissue damage and bleeding by sealing tissue, but the bleeding risk may vary depending on the measurement period. Previous studies have reported that hot dissection techniques such as coblation and bipolar diathermy scissor cause less intraoperative hemorrhage compared to cold steel dissection [18,27–29]. BiZact™ has also been reported to involve less intraoperative blood loss [15]. However, it has been reported that coblation and bipolar diathermy scissors have higher postoperative hemorrhage risks compared to cold steel dissection [10,30,31]. Hot dissection was also evaluated as having an increased risk of post-tonsillectomy bleeding compared to cold steel dissection [10,32–34]. The post-tonsillectomy bleeding risk of BiZact™ was reported to be around 0.16%–8.6% [5,12,16,35]. Meanwhile, overall post-tonsillectomy bleeding has been reported to be about 4.5% [11]. However, the bleeding risk may vary depending on the age and sex of the patient, as well as the indication for tonsillectomy, such as simple hypertrophied tonsil or recurrent tonsillitis [12,36]. Moreover, there is still no standardized measurement method for blood loss during tonsillectomy and no precise definition of post-tonsillectomy bleeding, so the accuracy of any such comparisons may be low [37].

In this study, postoperative pain after tonsillectomy using the BiZact™ device was not significantly reduced compared to the control group. BiZact™ can reduce tissue damage caused by heat by automatically controlling the energy delivered to tissues and sealing denatured proteins [12,38]. On the other hand, bipolar cauterization seals blood vessels and creates a thrombus, and Ligasure™ generates heat in short, delayed bursts to stop bleeding. Pain may occur due to inadvertent damage to soft tissue from thermal spread [5]. Therefore, it would be ideal to have a device for tonsillectomy that shows high hemostasis with minimal thermal damage [39]. However, it is not yet clear whether such tissue damage caused by heat is directly related to post-tonsillectomy pain [40]. In previous studies, bipolar cauterization or the radiofrequency technique were shown to cause reduced or similar pain compared with cold steel dissection [40]. Tonsillectomy using coblation has a tendency to cause less pain, but there may be differences in the pain assessment methods [27]. The age and gender of the target patients and the surgeon's skill level may have an impact on post-tonsillectomy pain [41–43]. A previous study reported that the return rates of patients who were operated on using the BiZact™ device were lower than those who were operated on through coblation, and this should also be considered [16].

Because the BiZact™ device uses a disposable handpiece, the cost of the technique using this device is higher than that of cold steel dissection. While the bipolar technique costs about USD 30, the BiZact™ technique costs about USD 275, which is about nine times that of the bipolar technique [17]. However, the high cost can be offset by the significantly shorter intraoperative time of BiZact™, which is approximately nine times shorter. BiZact™, which reduces operating room costs, can also be expected to have a long-term cost-saving effect [5]. However, comprehensive cost-effectiveness must be evaluated by comparing the long-term outcome and other complications of tonsillectomy.

This study also had some limitations that should be noted. First, several of the included studies were retrospective studies. There may therefore have been missing information on post-tonsillectomy pain and bleeding in the chart reviews of retrospective studies. Further prospective studies evaluating differences in bleeding risk and post-tonsillectomy pain should thus be included. Second, post-tonsillectomy pain was assessed by different clinics and researchers in each study, and it may have been influenced by the analgesics used during and after tonsillectomy. Third, bleeding risk may vary from study to study. There is a need for a prospective study using the same method for measuring intraoperative blood loss and the exact definition of post-tonsillectomy bleeding. Fourth, the surgical methods used may vary depending on the study. There may be efforts to reduce pain by reducing thermal injury through saline irrigation during tonsillectomy, or attempts to reduce bleeding through local injection. Alternatively, bipolar cauterization may have been used to reduce bleeding. In addition, Besser et al. performed BiZact™ tonsillectomy on one tonsil and cold-steel tonsillectomy on the other tonsil (control group) of the same patients and evaluated the outcomes differently, but the control group may have been different from other studies. Fifth, cold-steel dissection tonsillectomy is not clinically completely classified from bipolar tonsillectomy because it partially uses localized bipolar cauterization. Sixth, it cannot be ruled out that patients used other oral or topical medications for pain control before or after treatment that were not recorded in the medical charts. Lastly, bias related to the funding used in the few studies using BiZact™ is another potential problem. There is a need for additional research without industry sponsorship or any conflicts of interest.

5. Conclusions

The BiZact™ device for tonsillectomy significantly reduced operating time, but it was not superior in effectively reducing intraoperative bleeding, postoperative pain, or bleeding. It is necessary to compare the long-term results and additional surgical complications to comprehensively assess cost-effectiveness.

Supplementary Materials: The following supporting information can be downloaded at: https://www.mdpi.com/article/10.3390/medicina60091415/s1, Table S1: Quality of individual randomized controlled trial methodology; Table S2: Quality of individual non-randomized controlled trial methodology.

Author Contributions: Conceptualization: S.H.H.; Data curation: G.S. and Y.J.K.; Formal analysis: S.H.H.; Funding acquisition: S.H.H. and Y.J.K.; Methodology: S.H.H. and G.S.; Project administration: S.H.H.; Visualization: S.H.H.; Writing—original draft: Y.J.K. and S.H.H.; Writing—review and editing: Y.J.K. and G.S. All authors have read and agreed to the published version of the manuscript.

Funding: This work was supported by a National Research Foundation of Korea (NRF) grant funded by the Korean government (MSIT) (2022R1F1A1066232). And this work was supported by the Soonchunhyang University Research Fund. The sponsors had no role in the study design, data collection and analysis, decision to publish, or preparation of the manuscript.

Institutional Review Board Statement: Not applicable.

Informed Consent Statement: Not applicable.

Data Availability Statement: The raw data of individual articles used in this meta-analysis are included in the main text or Supplementary data.

Conflicts of Interest: The authors declare no conflicts of interest.

References

1. Manhein, D.; Raeder, J. Comparison of Bizact™ Low Temperature Dissecting Device with Bipolar Diathermic Scissors for Tonsillectomy in Adult Patients. *Austin. J. Surg.* **2023**, *10*, 1300. [CrossRef]
2. Younis, R.T.; Lazar, R.H. History and current practice of tonsillectomy. *Laryngoscope* **2002**, *112*, 3–5. [CrossRef] [PubMed]
3. Aldamluji, N.; Burgess, A.; Pogatzki-Zahn, E.; Raeder, J.; Beloeil, H. PROSPECT guideline for tonsillectomy: Systematic review and procedure-specific postoperative pain management recommendations. *Anaesthesia* **2021**, *76*, 947–961. [CrossRef]
4. Warnock, F.F.; Lander, J. Pain progression, intensity and outcomes following tonsillectomy. *Pain* **1998**, *75*, 37–45. [CrossRef]
5. Chuang, F.; Jones, R.; Quail, G.; Whitfield, B.; Ahluwalia, S. Rates of post-tonsillectomy haemorrhage between BiZact TM and bipolar tonsillectomy—A retrospective study. *Aust. J. Otolaryngol.* **2024**, *7*, 5. [CrossRef]
6. Arbin, L.; Enlund, M.; Knutsson, J. Post-tonsillectomy pain after using bipolar diathermy scissors or the harmonic scalpel: A randomised blinded study. *Eur. Arch. Otorhinolaryngol.* **2017**, *274*, 2281–2285. [CrossRef] [PubMed]
7. Ozkiriş, M.; Kapusuz, Z.; Saydam, L. Comparison of three techniques in adult tonsillectomy. *Eur. Arch. Otorhinolaryngol.* **2013**, *270*, 1143–1147. [CrossRef]
8. Ragab, S.M. Six years of evidence-based adult dissection tonsillectomy with ultrasonic scalpel, bipolar electrocautery, bipolar radiofrequency or 'cold steel' dissection. *J. Laryngol. Otol.* **2012**, *126*, 1056–1062. [CrossRef] [PubMed]
9. Worthington, T.C. A simple method of excision of the faucial tonsil. *J. Am. Med. Assoc.* **1907**, *48*, 1761–1762. [CrossRef]

10. Lowe, D.; van der Meulen, J.; Cromwell, D.; Lewsey, J.; Copley, L.; Browne, J.; Yung, M.; Brown, P. Key messages from the National Prospective Tonsillectomy Audit. *Laryngoscope* **2007**, *117*, 717–724. [CrossRef]
11. Blakley, B.W. Post-tonsillectomy bleeding: How much is too much? *Otolaryngol. Head Neck Surg.* **2009**, *140*, 288–290. [CrossRef] [PubMed]
12. Falz, H.; von Lücken, H.J.; Münscher, A.; Möckelmann, N. A comparative study of BiZact™ tonsillectomy versus cold steel dissection technique in adults: Analysis of operating time, intraoperative blood loss, postoperative bleeding rate and pain. *Clin. Otolaryngol.* **2024**, *49*, 299–305. [CrossRef]
13. Housley, D.M.; Imrie, J.; Low, C. Clinical utility of local over general anesthetic tonsillectomy using the BiZact™ device. *Am. J. Otolaryngol.* **2022**, *43*, 103547. [CrossRef] [PubMed]
14. Dulku, K.; Toll, E.; Kwun, J.; van der Meer, G. The learning curve of BiZact™ tonsillectomy. *Int. J. Pediatr. Otorhinolaryngol.* **2022**, *158*, 111155. [CrossRef]
15. Krishnan, G.; Stepan, L.; Du, C.; Padhye, V.; Bassiouni, A.; Dharmawardana, N.; Ooi, E.H.; Krishnan, S. Tonsillectomy using the BiZact: A pilot study in 186 children and adults. *Clin. Otolaryngol.* **2019**, *44*, 392–396. [CrossRef] [PubMed]
16. Ni, G.; McAuliffe, D.; Sethi, H.K.; Patel, P.; Terk, A. A single center retrospective comparison of post-tonsillectomy hemorrhage between BiZact and Coblator. *Int. J. Pediatr. Otorhinolaryngol.* **2022**, *158*, 111165. [CrossRef]
17. Stepan, L.; Huang, L.; Huynh, J.; Xie, P.; Woods, C.M.; Ooi, E.H. Health Related Quality of Life T-14 Outcomes for Pediatric Bizact Tonsillectomy. *Medicina* **2021**, *57*, 480. [CrossRef]
18. Lachanas, V.A.; Prokopakis, E.P.; Bourolias, C.A.; Karatzanis, A.D.; Malandrakis, S.G.; Helidonis, E.S.; Velegrakis, G.A. Ligasure versus cold knife tonsillectomy. *Laryngoscope* **2005**, *115*, 1591–1594. [CrossRef]
19. Page, M.J.; McKenzie, J.E.; Bossuyt, P.M.; Boutron, I.; Hoffmann, T.C.; Mulrow, C.D.; Shamseer, L.; Tetzlaff, J.M.; Akl, E.A.; Brennan, S.E.; et al. The PRISMA 2020 statement: An updated guideline for reporting systematic reviews. *Syst. Rev.* **2021**, *10*, 89. [CrossRef]
20. Besser, G.; Grasl, S.; Meyer, E.L.; Schnoell, J.; Bartosik, T.J.; Brkic, F.F.; Heiduschka, G. A novel electrosurgical divider: Performance in a self-controlled tonsillectomy study. *Eur. Arch. Otorhinolaryngol.* **2022**, *279*, 2109–2115. [CrossRef]
21. Saleem, M.; Alamgir, A.; Ali, S.J.; Hyder, H.S.; Bibi, S.; Saleem, S.T.; Alamgir, A.; Ali, S.J.; Hyder, H.S.; Bibi, S.; et al. Conventional Cold steel and Modern technique BiZact LigaSure for tonsillectomy: A comparative analysis. *J. Rawalpindi Med. Coll.* **2022**, *26*, 253–256. [CrossRef]
22. Yavuz Sultan Selim Yıldırım, O.S. Comparison of Bizact™ and Bipolar Tonsillectomy in Pediatric Patients. *SAS J. Med.* **2023**, *9*, 984–988. [CrossRef]
23. Kang, Y.J.; Stybayeva, G.; Hwang, S.H. Effects of glossopharyngeal nerve block on pain control after tonsillectomy: A systemic review and meta-analysis. *ANZ J. Surg.* **2024**, *94*, 1021–1029. [CrossRef]
24. Loh, R.; Stepan, L.; Zhen, E.; Shaw, C.L. Argon plasma coagulation tonsillectomy versus coblation tonsillectomy: A comparison of efficacy and safety. *J. Laryngol. Otol.* **2019**, *133*, 520–525. [CrossRef] [PubMed]
25. Kirazli, T.; Bilgen, C.; Midilli, R.; Ogüt, F.; Uyar, M.; Kedek, A. Bipolar electrodissection tonsillectomy in children. *Eur. Arch. Otorhinolaryngol.* **2005**, *262*, 716–718. [CrossRef]
26. Kemal, O. Harmonic scalpel versus bipolar tonsillectomy: A double-blind clinical trial. *Eur. Arch. Otorhinolaryngol.* **2012**, *269*, 1533–1536. [CrossRef]
27. Metcalfe, C.; Muzaffar, J.; Daultrey, C.; Coulson, C. Coblation tonsillectomy: A systematic review and descriptive analysis. *Eur. Arch. Otorhinolaryngol.* **2017**, *274*, 2637–2647. [CrossRef]
28. Elbadawey, M.R.; Hegazy, H.M.; Eltahan, A.E.; Powell, J. A randomised controlled trial of coblation, diode laser and cold dissection in paediatric tonsillectomy. *J. Laryngol. Otol.* **2015**, *129*, 1058–1063. [CrossRef]
29. Dadgarnia, M.H.; Aghaei, M.A.; Atighechi, S.; Behniafard, N.; Vahidi, M.R.; Meybodian, M.; Zand, V.; Vajihinejad, M.; Ansari, A. The comparison of bleeding and pain after tonsillectomy in bipolar electrocautery vs cold dissection. *Int. J. Pediatr. Otorhinolaryngol.* **2016**, *89*, 38–41. [CrossRef] [PubMed]
30. Söderman, A.C.; Odhagen, E.; Ericsson, E.; Hemlin, C.; Hultcrantz, E.; Sunnergren, O.; Stalfors, J. Post-tonsillectomy haemorrhage rates are related to technique for dissection and for haemostasis. An analysis of 15734 patients in the National Tonsil Surgery Register in Sweden. *Clin. Otolaryngol.* **2015**, *40*, 248–254. [CrossRef]
31. Aydin, S.; Taskin, U.; Altas, B.; Erdil, M.; Senturk, T.; Celebi, S.; Oktay, M.F. Post-tonsillectomy morbidities: Randomised, prospective controlled clinical trial of cold dissection versus thermal welding tonsillectomy. *J. Laryngol. Otol.* **2014**, *128*, 163–165. [CrossRef] [PubMed]
32. Lowe, D.; van der Meulen, J. Tonsillectomy technique as a risk factor for postoperative haemorrhage. *Lancet* **2004**, *364*, 697–702.
33. Gendy, S.; O'Leary, M.; Colreavy, M.; Rowley, H.; O'Dwyer, T.; Blayney, A. Tonsillectomy–cold dissection vs. hot dissection: A prospective study. *Ir. Med. J.* **2005**, *98*, 243–244. [PubMed]
34. Lee, M.S.; Montague, M.L.; Hussain, S.S. Post-tonsillectomy hemorrhage: Cold versus hot dissection. *Otolaryngol. Head Neck Surg.* **2004**, *131*, 833–836. [CrossRef] [PubMed]
35. Hessén Söderman, A.C.; Ericsson, E.; Hemlin, C.; Hultcrantz, E.; Månsson, I.; Roos, K.; Stalfors, J. Reduced risk of primary postoperative hemorrhage after tonsil surgery in Sweden: Results from the National Tonsil Surgery Register in Sweden covering more than 10 years and 54,696 operations. *Laryngoscope* **2011**, *121*, 2322–2326. [CrossRef]

36. Ikoma, R.; Sakane, S.; Niwa, K.; Kanetaka, S.; Kawano, T.; Oridate, N. Risk factors for post-tonsillectomy hemorrhage. *Auris Nasus Larynx.* **2014**, *41*, 376–379. [CrossRef]
37. Gysin, C.; Dulguerov, P. Hemorrhage after tonsillectomy: Does the surgical technique really matter? *ORL J. Otorhinolaryngol. Relat. Spec.* **2013**, *75*, 123–132. [CrossRef]
38. Kennedy, J.S.; Stranahan, P.L.; Taylor, K.D.; Chandler, J.G. High-burst-strength, feedback-controlled bipolar vessel sealing. *Surg. Endosc.* **1998**, *12*, 876–878. [CrossRef]
39. Družijanić, N.; Pogorelić, Z.; Perko, Z.; Mrklić, I.; Tomić, S. Comparison of lateral thermal damage of the human peritoneum using monopolar diathermy, Harmonic scalpel and LigaSure. *Can. J. Surg.* **2012**, *55*, 317–321. [CrossRef]
40. Boğrul, M.F.; Ünal, A.; Yılmaz, F.; Sancaktar, M.E.; Bakırtaş, M. Comparison of two modern and conventional tonsillectomy techniques in terms of postoperative pain and collateral tissue damage. *Eur. Arch. Otorhinolaryngol.* **2019**, *276*, 2061–2067. [CrossRef]
41. Tomkinson, A.; Harrison, W.; Owens, D.; Harris, S.; McClure, V.; Temple, M. Risk factors for postoperative hemorrhage following tonsillectomy. *Laryngoscope* **2011**, *121*, 279–288. [CrossRef] [PubMed]
42. Li, J.C.; Forer, M.; Veivers, D. Reference rate for post-tonsillectomy haemorrhage in Australia-A 2000–2020 national hospital morbidity database analysis. *PLoS ONE* **2022**, *17*, e0273320. [CrossRef] [PubMed]
43. Mao, B.; Woods, C.M.; Athanasiadis, T.; MacFarlane, P.; Boase, S.; Joshi, H.; Wood, J.; Ooi, E.H. BiZact™ tonsillectomy: Predictive factors for post-tonsillectomy haemorrhage from a 1717 case series. *Clin. Otolaryngol.* **2023**, *48*, 672–679. [CrossRef] [PubMed]

MDPI AG
Grosspeteranlage 5
4052 Basel
Switzerland
Tel.: +41 61 683 77 34

Medicina Editorial Office
E-mail: medicina@mdpi.com
www.mdpi.com/journal/medicina

www.ingramcontent.com/pod-product-compliance
Lightning Source LLC
Chambersburg PA
CBHW042009260926
51850CB00020B/2940
9783725844777